401 Fitness

How to Save Fitness for Your Retirement

By Doychin Karshovski

401 Fitness

How to Save Fitness for Your Retirement

© 2018 Doychin Karshovski

For information, contact the author:
Doychin Karshovski
6639 Paxton Guinea Road
Loveland, OH 45140

513-238-9952

Trainer@Want2goFit.com

www.401Fit.com

Illustrations: Vincent Vergara Cardones

Dedicated to Dad.

You were a loving and supportive father all your life.

I miss you.

Table of Contents

Introduction

401 Fitness

How to Save Fitness for Your Retirement

In high school I used to write good stories and get credits without much effort. Thirty-five years later, living on a different continent, writing in not my mother's language is not coming without an effort.

One might wonder why I am doing this. What is new and so important that I have to say to the world? Why don't I just write a blog or post on Facebook whatever I have to say and get it off my chest?

In Bulgaria, we have this expression: "Nobody forgive good that hasn't been asked for!" What that means is that you might think that you are doing something good for someone, but that person might have a different understanding of what is good for him or may not be ready and will not appreciate whatever you are doing, making it a double waste of time and effort for everybody.

In my career as a personal trainer I have often been in a position to clearly see that I can help a person who doesn't even realize they have a problem. We are more likely to seek help for things that we want, not for things that we need.

For example: I met this guy who really wanted to run a marathon. To do so without an injury, he needed to lose weight, develop stamina and strength. To lose weight he needed to become healthier and change his lifestyle. He knew he needed to do those changes, but he didn't want them. He wanted to run a marathon. This is just an example of how we think. We have this nice picture of ourselves doing cool stuff like running a marathon and receiving all the attention and credit for crossing the finish line. What a great conversation starter: "I ran that marathon."

On the other hand, making lifestyle changes and losing weight can be a long and lonely process where there are no crowds to cheer us on. Most of the time you on your own. Every one of us has the ability to make such changes, but we often need help, encouragement and motivation. We have been gifted with the most unique tool—the ability to make choices and act. We always have choices.

In my interactions with clients (I don't call this work because it goes beyond the job description of a personal trainer or wellness coach), I always try to give them what they need. What they "want" can be used as a strong motivator to help people push through the obstacles on their path to the goal.

I started *Want2goFit* in 2008 as an instrument to help people achieve what they want in fitness. Our journeys always start with something that we "want." They begin with a desire to change, to improve, to "go" from one place to another place where we know we will feel and be better. The "want" is still one of the most powerful motivators.

Every so often in my practice I would suggest a course of actions that the person would benefit from, but those actions might not be very appealing, not very "cool." To make sure this course will take place and the necessary positive changes will be achieved, I have to "sell" those "not cool" actions together with something that the person wants.

You won't be surprised if I tell you that one of the most "wanted" things is to lose weight. There are many ways to lose weight and there is only one way that is right for you. That's the one that will be based on understanding *why* the extra weight accumulated in the first place. Our bodies are designed to be healthy and fit. There is always a reason if they are not. To get what we "want," we first "need" to get healthy and allow our body to return to its original healthy state.

If you are guessing that such interaction and work is not easy, you are right. There is a significant line between being able to see through people's problems and suggest practical behavioral fixes and being able to judge what you see on the surface and then put a label on it. Judging has become something bad in our everyday dictionary.

To judge: to form an opinion about something or someone after careful thought.

In my profession, knowledge and experience very often rely also on intuition. If used properly, intuition can significantly help through the process of developing solutions. To figure out the original reasons why the person has become unhealthy or unfit in the first place is one of the most exciting parts of my work, and that process naturally doesn't stop there. Identifying and pointing out the problem does not lead to its easy fix.

4

For example, if a person is smoking and having problems breathing while exercising, the "easy" fix is to quit smoking, right? Of course, it's not easy to quit smoking or positively change any other addiction that might be blocking our path to better health. Very often I need to go deeper to see why the addiction happened at the first place and what other factors are in play.

We humans are complicated systems that have been designed to function in synergy and balance. Changing one part of the system leads to changes in other parts. If we understand how that system works, we can predict those responses and design positive lifestyle changes. Most of the time, we can't see our problems or even detect that we have one. We need an honest, critical, outside look at our history and behavior to figure out the best way to establish a healthy habit or get fit.

Many years ago, my very first official job was as a lifeguard on a very busy beach. I had been trained to constantly count the heads of the swimmers in front of me. When there was a missing head, that usually meant someone was in trouble and I had to rush to help and often save a life. There was no time to judge or form an opinion about that person's swimming skills. It was simple: A person needed immediate help and I was in a position to help. So I did!

One day there was a guy who came to swim when we were about to leave for the day. The sea was pretty rough. I had spent the whole day preventing people from getting in, and helping those who entered anyway to get back out of the water safely. I tried to talk the guy out of going for a swim, but he went in anyway. To cut this story short, I will only say it wasn't a pretty talk with that guy.

I decided to stay on the beach until he got out. His wife was waiting with me, obviously embarrassed by her husband's actions. She kept apologizing and telling me that he was a very good swimmer. Long story short—the guy started drowning and waving his hands. I rushed to help him, but his wife tried to stop me, telling me that he was waving just to say hi and that he was okay. I didn't even slow down.

It took me and my partner fifteen minutes to take this big guy out of the water. We used a rope back then: One of the lifeguards would swim with the rope as fast as he could to the drowning person. The rope was wrapped around the lifeguard's shoulders and he would grab the person from behind and hold his head above the water while the other lifeguard pulled them both out with the rope. The sandy rope would cut easily through skin and all the lifeguards had deep, bloody bruises for the whole summer.

Very often, people on the beach would come to help pull the rope. That day our "swimmer" was so tired it took him a while to catch his breath. The first thing he said was, "It wasn't necessary to pull me out, I was going to make it on my own." Back then I wasn't the nice, calm guy I am now. I will spare you my response.

I am telling you this story as an example to show that often we do not realize that we have a problem, even if it might be life-threatening. The people who are closest to us also might not see or might not want to point out that we have a problem. And of course, there is also that pride in every one of us that prevents us from asking for help. We tend to have this "happy ending" picture in our minds that everything will be okay on our own, and we don't need help. Well, sadly, very often we are not even qualified to recognize the needs we have. If someone suggests that we have a problem, we probably will take offense about being "judged." Even if we deep inside feel that he might be right.

Truth is, if we really need help we most likely will not make it on our own!

Even today, when I am on the beach or at a swimming pool I catch myself sitting with my face to the water and counting heads. Why I still do this? Because I know if somebody is drowning I can help.

7

In a way, I feel the same about writing this book.

If reading it helps you take actions and invest in your long-term health and fitness, I would be happy that I went through the process of writing it.

The idea for *401 Fitness* came to me at a lunch with my personal financial advisor and close friend Judy. While Judy was trying to explain to my confused fitness brain how 401-K and IRA work, I was wondering if there was a way to apply the simplicity and the mathematical logic of the long-term savings for financial retirement, and use those same principles to help people plan for staying healthy and fit.

I fully confess that while Judy was talking about my financial portfolio, I was shaping out my idea of *401 Fitness*. The idea kept growing in me. I was talking with my clients and friends, asking about their plans to stay healthy and fit in a long term. I also shared the concept with other fitness and wellness professionals. The vital interest and positive responses gave me the inspiration to develop the concept and put it in this book.

Good writing is always about something. This book is about the necessary minimum of movements, exercises and activities that we need in our everyday life to make sure we preserve our best physical mobility and autonomy as long as we live.

Here are few things this book will focus on:

1. Most people do not have long-term plans for staying fit. Many people don't have even short-term plans. Make a plan, see it through—we all know about this rule. If we don't have a plan we are not likely to accomplish our goals!

2. Another problem: If we are already active and have a plan to exercise regularly, we tend to focus on just one or two activities—most of the time just one. Yes, I know everybody has a favorite activity or sport. I love to swim and windsurf. Many of my clients run marathons and ride bikes. It is rare to meet somebody who has more than three different activities in his regular schedule. In the world of financial investment, that would mean that you haven't diversified your portfolio. Your investments are exposed to greater risk, and if the market moves unfavorably you might lose all of it. For fitness, the effect is similar. Imagine you are a runner that occasionally rides a bike and lifts weights. What would happen if you injured your ankle and can't run or bike or lift weights? Most likely you might stay inactive until you recover. The more we age, the more

time our body needs to recover. We do not have the "luxury" to be inactive at any time. Now imagine if you knew how to swim—you can still swim or do aqua aerobics and other activities in the pool while you are waiting for the ankle to heal, right? My point is that the more activities and skills we learn, the more choices we will have when limitations arise. By "diversifying" your fitness portfolio you will keep your fitness investments at low risk.

If we diversify our activities and get good at a wide variety of fitness, cardio, yoga and Pilates, if we learn to swim, play tennis, and sail a boat, we will have a great variety to ways to stay active. Also, the variety would greatly benefit our physical autonomy. It is definitely more fun and that makes it more likely we will stick to the plan and stay active and happy.

"Investing" in your fitness requires your personal time. No matter how much money you are paying for the latest equipment or gym membership or celebrity trainers, there is still no way of getting results without you personally showing up to do the work.

No trainer can do the work instead of you!

Wellness Concierge: the foundation of 401 Fitness

I have always been a big supporter of the notion that we need to keep trying new things and learning new skills. Apart from the obvious health benefits for the mind and body, this approach seems also to be more fun than to focus on only one or two activities. Nowadays, everywhere we go there are multiple options to exercise.

You can go to group fitness classes, lift weights or do yoga. The fitness industry is so diverse that even professionals like me have a hard time keeping up with the latest new choices and trends. Another thing that is very important for the success is a good match with the provider. We all have been there, when we have that favorite yoga teacher and we see that we perform and get the most from the teaching. How the personality of the instructor and that of the trainee match and sync is a very important element of a client's progress. It is also one of the best motivational resources for the trainer.

When was the last time you went to a class when you didn't like the trainer?

Thankfully, with the vast variety of trainers, teachers, classes and programs, we now have a great opportunity to find the perfect match. But this variety and the abundance of offerings can also be very frustrating, especially for beginners.

What if we had a way to utilize those vast resources and rich varieties of personalities, to map them and find a perfect match for every individual?

With this in mind, I started collecting and organizing information about all available fitness and wellness services in the Cincinnati area. For the past two years I attended hundreds of classes, met with trainers and teachers and explored exercise facilities.

I was blown away by the variety and the density of the available fitness resources. Every hour of the day, gyms offer classes, personal trainers are available for small groups or one-to-one training, and yoga studios have all kind of classes. And I am not talking yet about the ocean of online classes and one-on-one training out there.

To navigate through all this information and pick something that is right for you that matches your personality and fitness level with a specific trainer sounded like a difficult task. How could I make all this information available to help people get the right resource and be efficient in their efforts to be healthy and fit?

I tried a couple of different models and that is how *The Wellness Concierge* service was born. Why concierge? Because, as we know, the concierge always puts the client's needs first, to provide quality services of all kinds. Another reason I choose the *Wellness Concierge* title was to separate it from stereotypes of a "trainer" and a "coach."

It works this way: I meet with a client in person or online. We discuss their "needs" and "wants," and most importantly, personal availability and budget. During this process I take notes about their personality, fitness level and exercise history.

When I have all this information, I dig into my maps, studio list, class descriptions and teachers' bios and pick the ones that would work best for my client. Then I sit down and design a one-year plan that relies on services provided directly from me, and also on services that I know the client will benefit from, that are conveniently located and available according to the client's schedule.

I just described in a few sentences many hours of hard work, consultations, scheduling and personality matching, rate negotiations and other services. To make my efforts count I request at least a one-year commitment to the plan.

When the plan is confirmed, the only thing the client will need for the next year is to show up!

Remember, we talked about how that is the one thing we can't do for somebody else. So, we take care of the schedule, providing a variety of fitness and wellness services. We pick the classes and teachers to match a client's personality and fitness level, and we do the registration, so the client only needs to show up.

The goal is to help people establish a healthy and independent lifestyle. Clients also learn to maintain and heal their body and mind with simple daily exercises.

As great as this sounds, *The Wellness Concierge* has its flaws. First, it is not cheap. But the biggest investment is at the beginning. The more you follow the plan, learn new skills and adopt new activities, the less "intervention" from me you will see. If everything goes by the plan, in two years you should be able to continue on your own using the blueprint provided by me. You will have the skills, the fitness and the confidence to continue exercising on your own or use resources available in your surrounding area.

The second flaw of this service is that it is limited to just a small number of people.

You don't need to be a business expert to see that this is not a money-making model. We are not talking about retaining clients, we are talking about helping people to establish healthy and happy lifestyles. Ever since I started the *Wellness Concierge* I was thinking how I can make it more affordable and available for a wider group of people.

This book is my effort to bring that premium program to a wider group of people.

401 Fitness is based on the same understanding about the most important and fundamental activities that everyone should do to stay healthy and happy for life.

Part One

Chapter One

What We Were Made Of

Be humble for you are made of dung. Be noble for you are made of stars.

—Serbian proverb

Our physical and mental fitness affects our entire life and especially the last years of it. Paying attention and "investing" in our fitness ensures us not only against illnesses and injuries, but also sets us off on a long, healthy and happy life. When we are healthy we can focus on stuff that is important, like our family, career, art and community. If we are not healthy, the only thing that occupies our mind is how to get healthy, and that is how important health is for us. Being healthy allows us to live life in full, and that benefits all aspects of our society. Being healthy is always the first and most important element of happiness. Our bodies have been designed to be functional, balanced and healthy. When we put our bodies through challenges that push them out of balance, they adapt or get sick or both.

In the past hundred years science and technology have been rapidly changing our everyday life. We gladly accept all the benefits and perks that the new inventions bring in our lives. We are so used to having our entire world of friends right at our fingertips. We can ask any question and Google is very much likely to find an answer. Cars now run hundreds of miles on electricity. We have inhabited space with stations and satellites and now we are reaching for Mars.

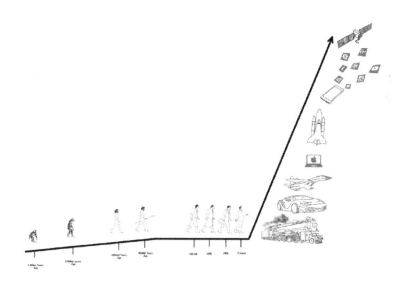

We can't even imagine life without computers, cell phones, GPS, Internet, drones. We have more technology in our pockets now than we used in the rocket that carried men to the Moon. And all these changes are happening so very fast. None of these inventions were around just fifty years ago. Yes, our bodies can adapt, but they can't do it this fast. They can't keep up with the speed at which science and technology change our environment. Our bodies haven't changed dramatically for thousands of years.

We know that our bodies can do amazing things. YouTube is full of unbelievable videos that prove our bodies can do amazing stuff. We cheer, share and comment about athletes, actors, dancers and even just next-door adventurers who take our breath away with their performances.

We are what we do. Have you heard that expression? We all have been equally designed to be healthy, strong, flexible, social. But at the end what we do every day is what it matters the most. We can become stronger, leaner and more flexible, or we can become a very efficient couch potato and let our well-designed body atrophy.

What we do every day matters. That is the blessing and the curse of our choice. We have the power to make decisions and the ability to act.

So, with our perfectly designed bodies and our unique ability to make choices and act, we should have everything under control, right? Then why are so many people today suffering from all kinds of diseases connected to stress, bad food choices and not enough movement? How come if we have the power to make good choices we end up sick, tired and unhappy? Is it possible to go back and revisit the blueprints of our body, understand how our bodies were designed to work and be maintained?

What if there is a way we can tap into those original blueprints and fix our health when we need to. There should be a way to stay healthy and fit even with the challenges of our fast-changing environment. We have the unique power to consciously choose our actions and by repeating them, establish habits that lead us to a healthy and happy state. We can easily adopt habits that make us sick; or we can adopt good habits that make us happy.

"We are what we repeatedly do. Excellence, then, is not an act, but a habit." -- Will Durant

Our actions and habits shape more than our bodies. It has been common knowledge for centuries that there is a connection between the mind and the body. The mind-body connection has been a goal for ancient martial arts systems, yoga and meditation. Now we have scientific evidence that every action we take affects our brain structure. Even thoughts that were believed to be immaterial are now proven to affect the matter of our bodies and shape our brain. Even more exciting is the discovery that those actions make their way all the way to our DNA, so what we do and think today can affect generations after us. How beautiful and kind of scary this responsibility is.

Knowing that with everything we do and think we shape not only our world but the world after us is a fascinating and very powerful motivator to do the right thing. But what is the right thing for us? What is the right thing for our bodies, for our minds, for our society? Seems like we might each have different answers to these questions, right? But what if we have some of the answers already pre-programmed in our DNA, in our bodies?

Our health and fitness are recorded in our original DNA blueprint. And we were designed to be healthy. Health is our natural state until our actions or the effect of our environment push us out of that balanced state. What if there is a way to tap into that DNA record and hit "reset" every time when we need to return to our healthy foundation? In his fascinating book *Pressing Reset: Original Strength Reloaded*, Tim Anderson maps out a unique program of original human movements that if done repeatedly (habitually) have the properties to reset our bodies and fitness to its original healthy state. The exercises and movements suggested by Tim are simple, and everyone should be able to do them. Tim's *Reset* system has been used by regular folks, people recovering from injuries and even professional athletes. It is fascinating to read through their amazing stories.

We were made to move and be strong. We were made to use our muscles and brains to interact with other people. What if there is a way to "maintain" our original strength to overcome the challenges of our busy schedules and long hours of sitting.

In the following chapter we will talk about the original movements and activities that are the most natural and beneficial to our bodies and minds.

Who wants to be a champion when he retires? That's what I thought: Even if there are some very athletic and competitive retirees out there, most of us envision retirement as pleasantly slowing down from all the craziness and stress. Playing golf, having lunch with friends and taking long vacations. If you are one of those who intend to run marathons and bike across the country after retirement, you can use this book and learn how to "save" even more fitness (mobility, stamina, range of motions), because you will definitely need it.

The rest who want to slow down and just enjoy an active and engaged life will find out that this book is not about six-pack abs and bench pressing twice your bodyweight. Instead, we will talk about how to choose your specific long-term fitness goals for retirement, how to make a plan and a budget to get there.

As with financial savings, the earlier you start, the more gain you will have in the long term.

Now ask yourself the following questions:

1. How many years do I have until retirement?
2. What are my main current health and fitness concerns?
3. What are my favorite fitness activities?
4. What would I like to do when I retire?

Answering these questions will help you get more from this book.

When you prepare for your financial retirement, the only thing you need is money that you can set aside and save or invest wisely so you can use the gains later when you need it. There are many ways we save money but this book is not about any of that. But there are similarities. When we talk about saving, setting aside valuable resources that we intend to use later, we think about discipline, planning, accountability, checks and balances and diversification of the investments.

All of these also apply to your fitness and health. The significant difference between money and fitness is that to save fitness you will always need your personal time.

We all have heard that saying, "I make money while I sleep"—usually from people who invested wisely and let their money grow without personal participation. Obviously, this is not an option when it comes to our fitness and health.

Being fit and healthy can be attained through simple daily exercises and balanced living

What is "working out" or exercising? Close your eyes and think about it for moment. What do you see? Ripped bodies, heavy weights and cardio machines?

If so, you are not alone! Exercise and fitness is a very visible and loud multibillion dollar industry that is everywhere around us, selling us something we "need" to get ripped, run faster or lift heavier weights. And this loudness is working. It puts a picture of the local gym or the

24

latest fitness gadget in our heads every time we think about working out. And of course, we know the price we need to pay. We pay with our time and our money, but they often will not match the image we have in our head for working out. Then we feel like we are losing the battle for our own health and fitness.

What if we change that fake picture in our heads?

According to *Webster's Dictionary*, a workout is "a practice or exercise to test or improve one's fitness for athletic competition, ability, or performance."

Did you notice that there is no mentioning of "belonging to a gym," buying a pair of running shoes or hiring a personal trainer?

So, if we get away from the fitness industry's selling noise, we should clearly see that the only things that we really need to work out (I personally like the term "exercise" better) is *our time and ourselves.*

Yes, some will say, "My time is the most precious thing and costs a lot of money!" I totally agree. That is why the whole concept of *401 Fitness* rests on small, time efficient fitness investments. We will talk about exercise blocks as short as five minutes, and focus on what is really important for the long term, with as little social sacrifice as possible. We will invest time to exercise, and time to develop relationships, as we discover what excites and inspires us.

We will start by determining what are the minimum physical abilities that we need to maintain to stay independent and active. Then we will expand that minimum, so the additional abilities and skills allow us to practice our favorite activities and maintain physical and social health.

Chapter 2

The Original Movements

Exercising our bodies and minds requires our full participation. The more mindful and connected we stay, the better results and joy we will get from our activities.

Since the beginning of our modern movement industry, fitness professionals have offered descriptions of the most fundamental human movements and exercises. The fundamental human movements are the ones that are the most natural to our bodies, involve our main muscle groups, and represent the way our body should move. Recognizing these movements, mastering their proper form and including them in our life would promote our health and prevent us from injuries in the long term. Here is a list of the five fundamental exercises that everyone should do, according to industry leader and Olympic weightlifter Dan John:

1. Squat
2. Push
3. Pull
4. Hinge
5. Carry

According to Dan, these exercises are the most essential in our everyday lives. If you look through your day you will probably discover all or some of these movement patterns. As you can see, sitting is not one of them.

In his book *Habitual Strength*, Tim Anderson suggests adding "Get Ups" to these five movements (a combination of the movements you do when you try to get up from the floor). I like that because even though you can see characteristics from the original five movements in the Get Ups, there are two very important "skills" that are not in the list described by Dan. If you try to get up from the floor in a smooth and efficient way you will discover how much *flexibility* and *balance* you possess. You will need strength to push your body weight off the floor and press with your legs to stand up, utilizing at least three of the original five (Push, Squat, Hinge). But also, you will need flexibility to properly position your legs under your body, and coordination to make everything work together so you keep your balance through the movement. Flexibility and balance are important properties of our bodies. Investing in just these two can make our body expressions bolder, more satisfying and fun.

Sometimes in my work I would ask a client to try to stand up from the floor while holding a glass of water above his head. If you want to try this, do it with a plastic cup, half full or even without the water at first. You would be surprised how many people would spill some water at their first attempts of this, although it looks easy at first glance. Do some Get Ups, and you will discover how flexible your knees, hips and shoulders are—or not—and how well you can balance and distribute your weight.

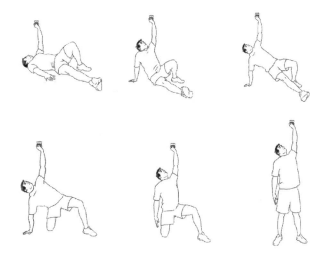

Another interesting list of original movements is suggested by Phil McDougall at the online health and fitness club *Strength Matters*. According to Phil, all daily movement and training programs should include the following seven patterns:

1. Locomotion

2. Hinge
3. Squat
4. Anti-rotation
5. Rotation
6. Push
7. Pull

The "new" additions in this list are Locomotion, Rotation and Anti-rotation. As Phil points out in his article, Locomotion "is the most important, but often neglected movement. It includes crawling, stepping up, walking, walking while carrying something, sprinting." Rotation and Anti-rotation include movements initiated or resisted in the torso.

There are many other professionals with their own suggestions for "must do" movements and exercises. The purpose of this book is not to give you yet another number of "must do" exercises, but to provide a smart tool that helps you to choose actions and put your efforts, time and money where you will receive the most fitness and health returns in a long term.

Fundamental movements are our natural way to preserve health and fitness. We know that we are supposed to be healthy and fit by design.

Health and fitness are hardwired deep in our bodies.

As Phil said in his article, "We all possessed almost perfect movement patterns as small children (before the chair and inactivity screwed everything up)."

Because we were designed to move naturally, it shouldn't be hard to re-establish the neural pathways that we were using when we first began moving. And the good news for all of us is that we can start from any point at any time and succeed.

This book is about recognizing the minimum of movements and activities that would ensure we age as healthy and independent human beings and enjoy an active and full life for our entire lifetimes.

This is not a book about bodybuilding and diets. This is a book that will help you choose your own minimum of activities that you need to stay healthy and fit—the way you were designed to be. Those movements and activities are the equivalent to *brushing your teeth every morning*—the minimum hygiene we need to promote our dental health.

Our bodies are unique systems that were designed to function in synchronization and balance, and respond and adapt to all the requests of our brains.

Our bodies are not machines! If you load a machine and repeatedly use it over and over at some point it will wear down, break or just stop. To keep the machines working we need to take constant care of them—apply grease here and there, change parts, balance elements...

What happens in our bodies if we use them over and over? Instead of wearing out, our bodies respond by adapting to the movements, loads and challenges that we throw at them. Our brain will discover the most efficient way for us to move and do the job, protecting us from breaking by developing stronger muscles and bones. The more we use our bodies, the better they become. Problems begin when we stop using moving and challenging the systems that were created to be challenged—our muscles, bones and brains.

Our unique body will respond to every order we give, even the ones that would lead to damages and even to death itself. If we say, "Stay on the couch and watch TV, eat chips and do not move at all," our body will comply. Our brain will actually try to make us "better" in those activities—because that is how we survived, adapted, got better and evolved. Asking our bodies over and over to adapt to sedentary habits is like a self-prescribed death sentence. Yet every day we see people choosing to live on that death row.

What we need to stay healthy, fit and sane is the constantly mindful use of our bodies and brain. Yes, it is that simple. But we have so many things to do and so many problems to care about and we don't have the time.

What if there is a magic "maintenance"—a minimum of "movement hygiene" that would prevent our bodies from going down that death road of atrophy?

What if we have this maintenance routine already hardwired in our human blueprint?

What if we can increase our chances of living long, healthy and happy lives with just few simple moves a day?

Here is my list of ten holistic human movements and activities that recover, revitalize and rebuild our neural pathways and maintain our original human strengths.

Breathing

Locomotion

Hinge

Squat

Rotation

Push

Pull

Brain Fitness

Social Fitness

Aqua Fitness

One of the biggest challenges for our health is sedentary life. There are many other factors that can make us sick and unhappy, but sedentary life is something that almost everyone has in common and it shouldn't be difficult to address and "fix" with proper lifestyle changes.

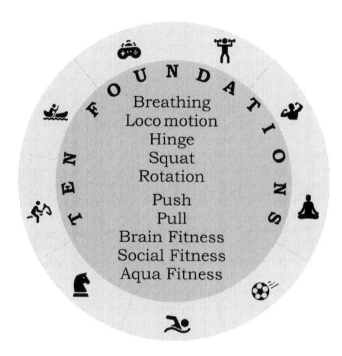

The movements and exercises presented in Diagram 1 (inside circle) can prevent and fight the negative effects of our modern sedentary lifestyle. To stay healthy and preserve fitness, everyone should have an amalgam of those *10 Holistic Exercises* in their daily routine.

As you can see, my list is a longer than the two

presented earlier. There are a few activities you won't see in a typical "fitness" program. My goal is to present a holistic tool: A *Wellness Blueprint*, that will help everybody to create his own fitness/wellness maintenance routine, to guarantee long and injury free functioning of our body and mind.

Let's first establish the role and the importance of every one of these activities.

Breathing

Without doubt, this is the one activity that is presented from our Day One to our last day on this earth. Breathing provides the air we need to function and there is nothing we can do without it. Breathing is deeply programed in our brain. We don't need to think about it; it is an instinct that automatically works for us. Any obstruction or slightest problem with our breathing would quickly disturb our health and can even lead to death. Even though it is an autonomic activity, we still have ways to control and modify our breathing:

- By the muscles we use to draw air in (diaphragm or chest)

- By the path we choose for inhaling and exhaling (nose or mouth)
- By the amount of air we inhale and exhale
- By the amount of time we inhale, exhale or hold our breath

The way we breathe affects not only our physical body, but also our psychological state of mind. Breathing has been described in ancient martial arts and yoga as the bridge between the mind and the body. Because we can control and use our breath to alter our body and mind, I put it in my list. We will talk about how in real life we can utilize breathing exercises in Part 3.

Locomotion

The ability to move our bodies from point A to point B has the most significance for us. It defines our independent life and our everyday functions. When we move from one place to another we use locomotor movements. Walking, crawling, running, hopping, skipping, jumping, leaping and galloping require that the spine and the trunk both are involved in producing and resisting dynamic forces.

A great example is crawling, when you place your hands on the ground and move forward, backward or to the side. When you crawl your normal orientation in space is changed. Your head is lower than your hips and that makes gravity to pull on your head and neck—great for relieving the tension that usually builds up there. The inversion also puts more work on your arms, shoulders and core, making them work in sync to move and maintain position.

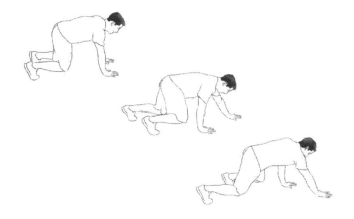

This simple challenge alone improves your upper spine, shoulders, and arm strength. In Part 3 we will talk about how to choose locomotor exercises to practice.

Hinge - Hips Don't Lie

When we talk about hinge in fitness, we mean a hinge in the hip. Often described as "the most fundamental movement," the hip hinge is not only a great move to build lower body strength but also protects your spine when you need to bend and lift stuff from the floor. Our sedentary life compromises the stability of our lumbar spine and the mobility of our thoracic spine. It is a recipe for back pain and even disability.

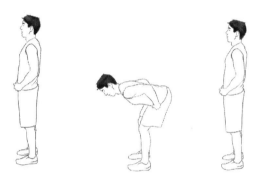

Maintaining our hip mobility, stability and strength is absolutely fundamental if we want to stay healthy and live an independent and happy life. One of the most popular exercises for training the hip hinge and the lower body is the deadlift.

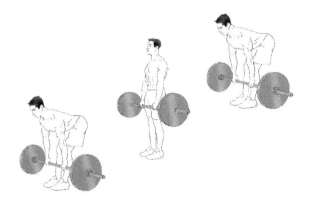

Squat

Have you seen a baby squat? It is amazing how smooth and effortless babies can just drop in a perfect squat and either stay there (a real challenge for most adults I know) or pick a toy and stand up. The squat is the ultimate test of flexibility and strength for our hips, back, knees and ankles. As an exercise, squats not only build lower body strength and flexibility, but also benefit our intestinal organs

Rotation

Rotation is movement in which something, e.g. a bone or a whole limb, pivots or revolves around a single long axis.

My *10 Holistic Exercises* includes torso rotation. The main function of the torso is to stabilize the spine and facilitate the movements initiated from the pelvic muscles. Torso is the "home" of the most famous "abs," or *rectus abdominus*, and also the less famous but not less important *transverse abdominis* and the *obliques*. Those are the primary muscles involved in a torso rotation movement.

Torso rotation also affects the rhomboids, deltoids, abductors, quads and adductors. Just the length of the list with muscles involved can be a reason enough to include torso rotation as a fundamental move. Exercising the torso benefits all the movements involving flexion, extension, and bending forward, backward and to the sides. The torso is also the distributing hub of all swinging movements and can significantly improve your performance in all sports that require swinging and throwing

Push

One of the most popular exercises is push-ups. Every time we move a load or weight away from our body—vertically or horizontally—we use a pushing motion. A very popular model of

41

401 Fitness

training is a push-pull routine that alternates pushing exercises with pulling exercises.

Pull

Similar to the push, this group of exercises represents movement of a load or weight in relation to the body. In this case, toward the body. Good examples are pull-ups, where the body weight represents the load that we are pulling vertically toward a mounted bar. Another example is rowing (horizontal), when we pull a load toward our body.

Brain Fitness

These are activities that challenge our abilities to solve problems and provide satisfactory feelings when we succeed. Both the challenge and the satisfactory feeling are very important for our brain health. Our life produces plenty of problems to be solved, but most of the time they might be complex and require a lot of time. Solving short, defined tasks provides the immediate rewards of satisfaction and joy of success that fuel up our brain and keep it healthy and fresh.

Examples are the "brain games"—puzzles, crossword, board games and so on. Our brain needs to play no less than our body needs to exercise. I can't stress enough the importance of our brain health! There is no way to be healthy, functional and happy if our brain is lazy and does not serve us well.

Brain Fitness is on my list to recognize the importance to keep the body and mind engaged and active.

Social Fitness

"No man is an island entire of itself; every man is a piece of the continent, a part of the main." -- John Donne

Social Fitness requires healthy, meaningful relationships with others. Our wellbeing is deeply dependent on our social interactions. This defines how healthy, trusted and valued our relationships are. The more we age, the more we need to be identified with social groups that provides us with meaningful interactions and relationships.

Relationships, friendships and affiliations are not easy to build and maintain. Over our lifetime we physically move from place to place. Changing work, neighborhoods and gyms can put us in a completely different social pool and disconnect us from the environment we are used to. Our interests, goals, social status and values also can change over time, and we might find ourselves in a social surrounding that no longer provides us with meaningful (for us) interactions and relationships.

Aqua Fitness

Under this category I put all exercises and movements that are performed in water, including but not only swimming.

Here are my reasons to include aqua fitness in my ten fitness foundations:

- Being in water is a very natural to us. It is easy to learn to float and move in water. I am not talking about swimming with perfect style breaststroke, backstroke, butterfly or even crawl. Just moving from point A to point B in water is a perfect whole-body exercise.
- We relax and relieve of stress naturally by just being in water.

■ If there is one activity that can combine the benefits from all the rest of the foundational exercises, that is swimming.

I also think swimming might be looked at as a locomotive activity like walking or crawling. I want to stress its significant importance for our health. If you swim you will cover at least five or six of the foundational movements. You have: 1. Breathing; 2. locomotion; 3. squat (when you push off the wall with both feet or swim breast stroke); 4. the pull (when you move your hands to propel your body forward); 5. rotation, and 6. anti-rotation (when your whole body responds to the multiple vectors of power and moves forward).

When I swim these days, I listen to music or audio books (what a great invention the waterproof iPod is!). I know it is a stretch to count this as a brain activity, but I often have found solutions and new ideas while I swim. My explanation is that when we get in the water we first must disconnect physically from our busy lives, then we get busy repeating natural movements in a safe and relaxing environment that our body and mind recognize. Without all the demands, our brain goes back to its original state of calmness. Ideas and solutions come easily to us while we swim and recharge our neural system.

If for any reason you haven't learned to swim, or float you should strongly consider doing so. You can start at any age and with any body type

Chapter Three

Never Too Old to be Fit

It's good to stay as close to real life as you can, and then kind of dress it up.

—Nelson DeMille

What is happening in real life actually can be quite different. If you take a look at your last week of activities and make a list, chances are it might look like mine here:

- Walking the dogs
- Writing this book
- Reading
- Playing Cards with friends
- Yoga
- Meditation
- Barre 3 class
- Swimming
- Windsurfing

We can easily match some of my activities with those in the circle of Ten Foundations presented before.

- Walking the dogs: This is clearly a locomotive exercise.
- Writing this book: Even though I write mostly in a deep squat and sitting and stretching on the floor, I would count writing as a brain fitness exercise.
- Reading: Brain fitness
- Playing Cards: Brain fitness
- **Yoga** Class
- Meditation: Breathing
- **Barre 3** Class
- Swimming: I swim laps every day, usually for at least 20 minutes, about a mile for that time, mostly free style
- **Windsurfing**

Let's say that we are living a life that has all the movements and activities from the Ten Foundations covered. Including those activities in our lifestyle should be enough for us to live long, healthy and autonomous life. But as you see from my list above there are so many other activities that are not "foundational"—we can't find them among the activities that are qualified as the Ten Foundations. What are those and why do we need them?

In my list, the activities in bold are without direct match to the Ten Foundations. Those are Windsurfing, Barre3 Class, and Yoga. These activities, together with many others, represent our outer circle of activities that I call "branded human activities," or just Branded Activities.

As you can see, that circle consists of activities that include and rely on the basic movements in our inner circle—on our foundation. By Branded Activities I mean those activities that were "human made." We recognize them by name, and when we hear the name (brand) we have a clear picture and understanding what they are. Some of them have been around for thousands of years, such as wrestling, hunting and yoga. Others are relatively new "brands," such as Barre3 classes, Pilates, soccer, football, curling, tennis...

Some are probably being "branded" while I am typing these words. These activities and sports are based on movement patterns and have rules that are supposed to challenge our bodies and minds. Some of them provide entertainment for spectators.

All Branded Activities are based on the Ten Foundations. There is no Branded Activity that doesn't involve at least one foundational movement. All sports are Branded Activities.

An interesting fact is that one of the first popular definitions of sport comes from England, where back in the days Boxing was considered as "the original sport." The bored rich English aristocrats with "sport spirit" used to say that sport is everything you can bet on.

All Branded Activities are "human made."

For the purpose of this book, I organize these activities in ten brands. Every brand should bring a picture in your head of at least one specific activity.

Branded Activities:

1. Body-weight activities: gymnastics, dancing, calisthenics, yoga, tai chi, martial arts
2. Activities with resistance: all weight liftings
3. Activities under time restriction: Interval training, Tabata, HIIT (high intensity interval training)
4. Sports with a ball: basketball, football, baseball, etc.
5. Sports with machines: car/truck racing, video computer games
6. Sports with animals: horse races, equestrian competition

7. Mind games: chess, cards, backgammon, puzzles, crosswords, Sudoku
8. Outdoor activities: hiking, camping, boating, hunting, photography, safari
9. Passive activities that directly benefit the body-mind connection: massage, body alignment, sauna, stretching, meditation, prayers, breathwork

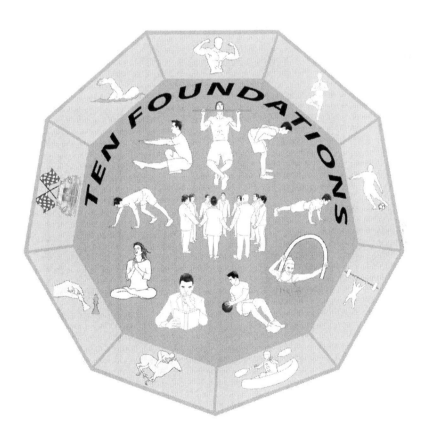

In this diagram, the inner circle contains the ten foundational activities that we established in Chapter Two. All Branded Activities are in the outer circle.

Our bodies are designed to move in many ways. We have the ability to perform complex activities by combining multiple foundational movements. Branded Activities represent the manifestation of our human body abilities. The list of the Branded Activities is constantly growing and developing with every new activity we choose to challenge our bodies with.

The ancient Olympic Games were initially a one-day event until 684 BC, when they were extended to three days. In the 5th century BC, the games were extended again to cover five days. The ancient games included running, long jump, shot put, javelin, boxing, pankration (an ancient Greek form of martial arts) and equestrian events.

Today we have Summer and Winter Olympic Games. The 2016 Summer Olympics included twenty-eight sports, with five additional sports due to be added to the 2020 Summer Olympics. The 2014 Winter Olympics included seven sports.

Getting personally involved (not just as a spectator) in sports and games and learning new activities from the Branded list is essential to our health and happiness. It provides us with an arena to test, explore and enjoy movement skills that we have developed in our Inner Circle of activities—the Ten Foundations. Getting involved in sports and other Branded Activities is also giving us an opportunity to apply and practice multiple foundational movements in a very efficient manner.

By engaging in multiple Branded Activities, we apply one of the most important principles from the financial world: *diversification.* The more diversified our fitness portfolio, the more different stocks (Branded Activities) we have in it, the more sustainable and less risky our (health) investments will be.

Translated to our health and fitness context, that means that *we need to constantly explore, learn and adopt new activities.* One of the reasons we need to do this is the problem I mentioned before. We tend to focus and stay mostly with just one activity. If we do more than one it is more likely from the same "brand." This is not sustainable in a long term and does not give our health and fitness the "best bang" for our time. For example, if your everyday activities include running and occasionally biking, and if one day you injure your ankle, you won't be able to do any of your familiar activities. What will happen is that you have to stop the activities that you have mastered and become inactive until you are healed. While you are healing you will be using your health savings—your body will use the stamina, the strength you have built exercising to heal your injury. The stronger you are, the more healing power your body will have to spend. At the end you will be healed but your health savings will be depleted. You need to start again and build up your stamina and strength slowly back to where they were. And that is actually the *happy* ending. Most of the time we never recover completely from injuries, especially if those are repeated injuries caused by the same activity over and over (tennis elbow, runner's knee, etc.).

We all have seen stories about great athletes who had to completely change their active lifestyle after an injury and lost the quality of life they had before. Their "health savings" has been used and they do not have other sources to build up their fitness again, because they invested in only one "stock"—their unique set of skills that they can't do anymore because of the injury. If you look at any physical therapy session you would notice that many foundational movements are being used, because the goal of PT is to help us recover our strength and full range of movements. Recovery is not building up fitness. Recovery is getting back to the basic foundation of our health. The building up happens when you invest your foundational skills in practicing (investing in) multiple Branded Activities from that second circle.

We can look at the inner circle as the minimum amount of money needed just to open your saving account. All the things shown in the outer circle are your options to "invest." It is a sad but true fact that many people haven't covered the ten holistic foundations in the inner circle yet. They jump in and "invest" heavy in some of the Branded Activities—the second circle. They can become very good and even perform at a professional level, but if they do not have the basics foundations covered and do not diversify in the second circle they can lose every gain the moment an injury happens.

Jennifer might be an excellent tennis player, but she will be sitting for weeks on the couch if she gets tennis elbow and has no other alternatives than playing tennis to stay fit. She has limited herself to one source of investment. And as we all know, injuries happen just as financial investments can have setbacks.

There is another reason why diversification of our fitness investments is so important. In our lives we learn skills, then use them through our active life to build a career, take care of our families and so on until retirement and the end of our lives. Dying is as natural as birth is. We all know of people who were not able to move or take care of themselves in their last years. Without the ability to perform any meaningful activity, those people were prisoners in their own still living bodies. The process of dying began the moment they were unable to perform their daily routine.

In his book *Live Long, Die Short: A Guide to Authentic Health and Successful Aging*, Dr. Roger Landry talks about "compression of morbidity"—meaning that the time we are sick at the end of our life is short.

Apart of viral or other diseases that we can catch at any time, if we maintain strong foundation of all the movements and abilities in the inner circle, our chances to have a long life and a short decline are better.

Jack LaLanne is the father of modern fitness and probably the most influential wellness figure of our times. He died in his sleep from bronchitis after a short illness at the age of 96. Until the last day of his life he was performing his usual daily exercises and enjoyed a full and active lifestyle.

How to live our life and how to die is in our hands. We can make lifestyle choices and invest in our health in a way to stretch our strength and physical abilities all the way to our last day.

The diagram below, represents the performance curve of a lifetime. The first part of the line is where we develop our physical abilities and learn new skills. The more we "invest" in that part, the higher our performance will be and the line will climb. The solid horizontal part of the line represents our years of best performance. The length of that period may vary depending on our line of work, it's intensity and our lifestyle. The more intense our work is, the shorter this line will be. A good example is professional athletes. The dashed line represents the "usual way" of our performance declining. This is the part of our life when we are losing performance and quality of life due to becoming weak, inactive, and sick. We used to blame age for all these losses.

But the historic McArthur Foundation study of Successful Aging proved that how we age is mostly up to us!

When we think about aging, we think about declining, giving away abilities, slowing down. The McArthur study proved that aging and declining are not necessarily connected by default. How we age is totally up to us. No, we can't change a lot of our environment, and social demands and challenges will always be part of our life. But at the end we have choices to make. We all have the same number of hours in our days. We have a choice to binge watch TV or go early to bed with a good book. We can sleep till it's time to jump in the car and rush for work, or we can wake up early to exercise and plan a healthy meal for the day.

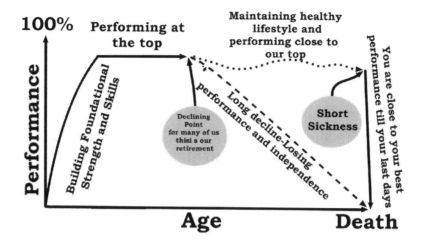

Every time we experience injury or sickness, our performance curve will be disrupted, and we will see a steep drop or a decline. But if our Ten Foundations are strong, that will be a short decline and we will regain quickly our strength and quality of life and our performance line will go up.

The orange line The curve dotted line represents the performance of a person who constantly invests in the Ten Foundations and stays active and engaged.

It's easy to build strength, endurance and the other components on a mobile body of any age.

Our lifestyle reflects not only our performance and quality of life but also the quality of our death. Who wants to spend his last years sick in bed with frequent visits to hospitals, with the need of constant care? Living a life dependent on the help of relatives, in constant pain and on medications, is not appealing to anybody. It is possible to live a long, healthy and happy life and avoid a long decline when the time comes.

Dr. Landry says, "As far as you put your honest effort in, it doesn't matter where you start. You will still have the positive outcome in the long run."

Below are Landry's suggestions for the main things to consider in order to age healthy and happy:

1. Minimize risk of disease and disability
2. Maintain physical and cognitive function
3. Keep your engagement with life, stay social and important

I like the simplicity of these suggestions. My goal with the Ten Foundations is to introduce specific activities that can be broken down to everyday tasks—small, doable tasks that allow us to invest in those areas that we need to improve our health or develop skills that will increase the quality of our life all the way to the end of our days.

Part Two

Chapter Four

Take Charge and Invest in Fitness

If you don't make the time to work on creating the life you want, you're eventually going to be forced to spend a LOT of time dealing with a life you DON'T want.

– Kevin Ngo

Take this self-evaluation quiz:

- Where am I with my fitness savings?
- What does my answer mean for me?
- What am I missing? How do I fix it?
- Why is this important?

Our health always reflects our lifestyle. When we are born, our health and wellbeing is based on our genetics, and the choices our parents made for their health during and before pregnancy.

At that first period of our life we are fully dependent and rely on lifestyle choices that our parents make for us. Growing up, we start to get more and more involved in the decisions about our life until the moment we are in full control. For me, that moment came when at age 18 I had to leave home and join the Army. In Bulgaria, every boy has to go in the Army after high school for two or three years depending, on if you are accepted in a college or not.

Like all my friends, I dreaded that moment and hoped to get an easy deployment or at least stay at the same city. At that time, I was in the Bulgarian National Marine Pentathlon team, as team captain for the second year. Marine Pentathlon is a sport that includes swimming, running, shooting at a target, rowing and sailing. The sport was under the umbrella of the Navy and we competed against teams from Eastern Europe. We also competed in underwater swimming, sailing and other individual disciplines. Most of my teammates and I got certified as professional scuba divers, and I also got a license as a captain of a seagoing vessel up to five hundred tons. At the age of 16, I became the youngest Master of Sport of Marine Pentathlon. Master of Sport is a lifetime recognition that got me accepted in college without exams and with full scholarship. So here I am at the age of 18 graduating from high school, already making money as a sailing and swimming coach, accepted by the best sports college in Europe with a girlfriend I have been in love with since ninth grade. Life wasn't looking very bad.

Well... "thanks" to my athletic background, I got a stamp as "Excellent Scuba Diver" in my military papers and was sent to serve one hundred miles away in a city where I didn't know anybody. So, at age 18 I was on my own, surviving in a very new and, to put it lightly, unfriendly environment. I am pretty sure the secret goal of my commanders and my senior Marines was to break us physically, mentally and socially.

I'll never forget the first forty-five days and the first year, when we "rookies" went through vigorous physical training, most of which would be better described as torture. When we were not in training we "enjoyed" mental and physical bullying, with constant deprivation of sleep and food.

Going back in that time now, I can clearly see choices that I made right and also those that have turned out not to be so good. Being young and arrogant, I took all my health, strength and stamina for granted. I am pretty sure I didn't even know the meaning of "holistic" or "wellness", but somehow, I subconsciously adopted lifestyle habits that were based on those concepts and are the foundation of my health now.

Just a few examples:

Starting out early in the morning was no fun at the beginning, especially when instead of an alarm clock you got a bucket of ice cold water to wake you up. But now, thirty years later, I appreciate the calmness and the creativity that my early morning hours give me.

Eating in the Army was a time that you wouldn't think can be tough, right? Well, now imagine if you are given five minutes to eat, in which time you are constantly grilled with questions about the Navy rules or asked to disassemble or assemble any type of weapons on the table. Oh, and you need to stand at "attention" every time somebody with more seniority says your name. Sounds like a lot of fun, right? I learned to appreciate my time for eating and especially chewing. Today, I always take my time to set my table and enjoy every meal. I appreciate where the food came from and how it was prepared.

Many of my fellow Marines were also professional athletes in different sports. I remember a guy who was a great Olympic weightlifter. He was having a very hard time with all the running we had to do and I had to keep an eye for him all the time during water exercises. I learned to appreciate my versatile skills and abilities and worked to develop them even further.

One of my most valuable lessons from that time wasn't related to physical activities. I discovered how much my happiness depends on being with people that I like spending quality time with. For two years I had only twenty days of release that I was able to go home. This is the era before internet and cell phones. I discovered how writing can keep my sanity. I wasn't big in journaling, but I was using every quiet moment to write letters to my parents, my coach, and of course to my girlfriend. These and other choices I made back then helped me to survive that period, gain confidence in my abilities to be in charge in my own life.

It doesn't matter when or where we take charge of ourselves and become aware of the decisions we make and their effect on our health and wellness. We all have the same power of making choices that shape our life. Every choice counts and whether we realize it or not, we are constantly shaping our health and life. Realizing that we are in control is a very important moment for our wellbeing.

I see people every day that even though being adults, making money and independently living have not acknowledged and more importantly have not utilized the power of making choices. Every decision we make affects our health/fitness account. We either add to gain health, or we pay with the health "savings" we already have. But what choices to make and how to make sure they will be good for us?

Let's assume that at birth we all get a clean health credit. When we become grownups and have to take control of our own health, we already have been exposed to many ups and downs. Our health/fitness credit score might not be perfect any more. Our health foundations might be poor or not developed at all. Most likely we will have missing or neglected bricks in our Ten Foundations.

In this chapter we will talk about how to self-evaluate your Ten Foundations and how to choose lifestyle changes that will build up your health/fitness credit—your health foundation. Once we get the Ten Foundations covered, we will explore how to invest our fitness capital into Branded Activities that will guarantee sustainable growth and increase our chances to live long and health until the end of our lives.

Let's take a look at our Ten Foundations: Breathing, Locomotion, Hinge, Squat, Rotation, Push, Pull, Brain Fitness, Social Fitness and Aqua Fitness. Unless you are training for the Bulgarian Marine Pentathlon, it is not possible and it is not efficient to include all of these in a single day. The good thing is that our daily routines probably already include some of those. Remember my list of activities and how we were able to match some of the activities with the Ten Foundations and the rest with the Branded Activities? The purpose of the following quiz is to help you find out which foundations you have covered in your established routine and which you need to work on.

But what if you discover from the quiz that you walk only to and from your car—is that enough to mark the Locomotion foundation covered? Or Breathing, for example: of course, we have to breathe constantly. Can we check off that foundation? How much is enough? If you do just one squat during the day, can you claim that you have that movement covered?

To evaluate how the basic movements and activities are represented in our everyday life, I suggest the following quiz. Here are few important points to consider when answering the questions:

All practices, movements and activities should be easily recognized in your everyday routine as stand-alone activities, or as part of a more complex daily activity. In my own list, walking the dogs is easily recognized as Locomotion, but attending a yoga class can be many things that fit the description of one or more of the Ten Foundations. In my yoga class we usually do twenty or thirty Vinyasa Flow movements that can be easily recognized as a form of push up (Push foundation).

Here is what I suggest as "qualifying" repetitions and lengths:

Breath Work: breathing exercises, singing out loud, or giving a speech or a lecture.

At least five minutes of uninterrupted practice.

Locomotion: crawling, stepping up, walking, walking while carrying weight, sprinting.

At least five minutes of uninterrupted practice.

Hinge: bending over, bridge, deadlift.

One - two minutes of uninterrupted activity that includes those movements.

Squat: squat on flat feet, rocking, single leg squats, goblet squats, hold squat, chair pose in yoga.

One - two minutes of uninterrupted activity that includes those movements.

Rotation: reaching, throwing, boxing, windmill and opposite anti-rotation, as with single-arm or single-leg resistance training.

One - two minutes of uninterrupted activity that includes those movements.

Push: press in all directions, push-up, a dip or military press.

One - two minutes of uninterrupted activity that includes those movements.

Pull: pull in all directions, pulling yourself up onto something, climbing.

One - two minutes of uninterrupted activity that includes those movements.

Brain games: chess, backgammon, puzzles, Sudoku, crosswords, active reading, creative writing.

At least twenty minutes of brain stimulating activities daily.

Social Fitness: meetups, affiliations, volunteer work, etc. Actual activities should be presented—not just a membership.

One to two hours of engagement every month.

Aqua Fitness: water walk, floating, swimming strokes.

At least thirty minutes every month.

The first eight activities—Breathwork, Locomotion, Hinge, Squat, Rotation, Push, Pull, and Brain Fitness—should be done every single day. The other two—Social Fitness and Aqua Fitness—should be covered in a month.

The goal of the quiz is to figure out how much of the Ten Foundations you are covering with your daily routine. Keeping this in mind, answer the following questions.

Quiz

Circle the answer that best describes your activity.

1.   **Breath Work:** breathing exercises, singing out loud, giving a speech, swimming.

A. I do every day.

B. I do every week.

C. I do every month.

D. I don't remember doing it.

2. **Locomotion:** crawling, stepping up, walking, walking while carrying weight, sprinting.

A. I do every day.

B. I do every week.

C. I do every month.

D. I don't remember doing it.

3. **Hinge:** bending over, bridge, deadlift.

A. I do every day.

B. I do every week.

C. I do every month.

D. I don't remember doing it.

4. **Squat.**

A. I do every day.

B. I do every week.

C. I do every month.

D. I don't remember doing it.

5. **Rotation and Anti-rotation.**

A. I do every day.

B. I do every week.

C. I do every month.

D. I don't remember doing it.

6. **Push.**

A. I do every day.

B. I do every week.

C. I do every month.

D. I don't remember doing it.

7. **Pull.**

A. I do every day.

B. I do every week.

C. I do every month.

D. I don't remember doing it.

8. **Brain games:**

A. I do every day.

B. I do every week.

C. I do every month.

D. I don't remember doing it.

9. **Social Activities:** club memberships, meetups, affiliations, volunteer work.

A. I do every day.

B. I do every week.

C. I do every month.

D. I don't remember doing it.

10. **Aqua Fitness.**

A. I do every day.

B. I do every week.

C. I do every month.

D. I don't remember doing it.

Here are how much your answers are worth in fitness Coins—call it your fitness wage ("fitwage").

$$A = 50$$
$$B = 20$$
$$C = 0.5$$
$$D = 0$$

If you have answered with an A on the first eight questions and with A, B or C on the last two questions, you have your foundations covered.

So, if we have the requirements covered, our minimum score should be at least 401:

8x (A) 50 = 400

2x (C) 0.5 = 1

Minimum score = 401

Of course, right now you can be in good shape and health even with a lower score. The purpose of this test is to show your areas where you need to focus to get all your Ten Foundations covered and increase your chances to live a healthy and independent life.

Now imagine a game of Monopoly—every time you complete the circle you get two hundred dollars from the bank for passing "Go," right? For every <u>month</u> of your life that you get all your foundations covered, you get 401 Fitness "Coins" for passing Go. This is your fitness wage (fitwage). When you have your *fitness capital* built up you can invest it and save more fitness and health. Here is a simple formula to determine how much capital you need before starting to invest based on your answers:

If you have saved less than 401 fitness Coins, you need to invest in your missing foundations. If you have 401 or more, you can start to diversify your fitness portfolio and invest in activities that are new for you.

By building your fitness foundations you are increasing your health capital one fitness Coin at a time.

Here is another way to look at it: Let's imagine for a moment that the variety of activities you do represent your options to invest in the stock market. Your investment capital will be your current fitness and health based on your Ten Foundations and measured in Fitness Coins. You can invest that fitness capital in all kinds of stocks—those are your Branded Activities. The healthier you are, the more capital you have to invest. If you invest wisely, your health capital (Ten Foundations) will grow and your fitness and health will keep improving. There will be times when injuries or unpredicted circumstances would cause disturbances or even "crash" your fitness market, but if your investments have been consistent and your portfolio is balanced and diversified, you will survive the market turbulence and your original health capital won't be hurt.

As we see in diagram 1, the inner circle includes all the movement and activities we consider fundamental for our health in the Ten Foundations. How we can make this work in real life? How we can cover all the bases and make sure we are adding savings to our health and fitness, while we continue to invest in new skills and activities that will make us even healthier and stronger?

In order to further simplify these activities, I organized them in groups by their maintenance period—the minimum of time a single activity should be repeated for optimum health/fitness saving results.

Minimum Requirements for Maintenance of the Ten Foundations

Daily	Breathing	Locom.	Hinge	Squat	Pull	Push	Rotations	Brain Fitness
	5 min.	5 min.	1 min.	1 min.	1min.	1 min.	1 min.	10 min.
Monthly	Social Fitness 1- 2 hours					Aqua Fitness 30-45 min		

Chapter Five

Put Money in Perspective

Every cent you own and every moment you spend is always an investment.

—Natalie Pace

Being married for twenty-six years to an accountant (that same girl from the 9th grade that I wrote letters to), I have been exposed to many "accounting" talks at our dinner table that made me appreciate the science and art behind the terms and the numbers.

For the most of us, accounting is boring but accurate system of rules to track and report expenses. I would like to further simplify this sophisticated and complex system and invite you to look at it in a new way. Imagine that you have only two columns in your Fitness Balance Sheet to track every fitness "transaction"—a column named Give (In) and a column called Take (Out):

Give to your health	Take out of your health
Walking the dogs	Sitting for long hours
Stretching	Smoking

Every action we take can apply to one of this two columns in our fitness account. It will be either a Take (from our health) or a Give (being good to our health and fitness).

For example, a walk in the park goes into the Give column. But three hours of binge watching TV definitely goes into your Take column.

Every action and every decision we make, even the most complex ones, can be split and sorted into these two categories. The reason I offer this perspective is to help you know and understand where your actions fall. That will help you take ownership of your own decisions and be a better judge of what is good and what is bad for you.

Here our Ten Foundations and Branded Activities come in very handy. They are easy to

81

recognize in our daily life and, of course, they belong in the Give column, because they bring value to our health and build our wellness capital.

Other activities that are not so easy to recognize as a Give or a Take can be broken down until we see how they fit on our fitness balance sheet. For example, working on a crossword puzzle in the newspaper while eating a donut can be split into two activities—one that matches one of our Ten Foundations and is good for our health, and one that is easily categorized as destroying our health. If you can guess which is which, you already have been doing your own health accounting. Congratulations!

Now test your new accounting skills on *walking in the park while smoking a cigarette.*

We can't always choose activities that are only good for us. Our lives constantly demand expenses from our fitness savings. That's OK as long as we are aware of it. I do not picture myself or anybody else walking around with a fitness balance spreadsheet all day long, while consciously classifying every activity in the proper column. We just need to be aware of this process of constant exchange that is happening in every moment of our lives.

Knowing that our actions will always fall into one of these categories can be a great self-motivation tool for the lifestyle changes we intend to accomplish.

On the other hand, if you decide to actually keep a record of your actions and activities for a certain period of time, you might notice patterns that have escaped your attention. By identifying them you will be in a better position to choose positive lifestyle changes.

Making a positive change in your life can start with a simple addition to your Give column or subtracting an action that has been a longtime health drain in your Take column. The power of making choices is always at your disposal. Use it. There are so many ways.

Suppose you know that you will sit in traffic for the next hour. You can't avoid this health expense, because it is necessary to go to work and provide for your family. But you have the power of adding a little to your Give column to balance your health expense. Pick a good audio book or a podcast, for example, or make sure you keep that massage appointment that you have been rescheduling. Pay something back to your health account.

If we look at people on the street we are not likely to recognize who owes money to IRS or has maxed out their credit cards or filed for bankruptcy. Those events do not affect the way we look and our health, at least not on the surface. But numerous studies suggest that our physical and mental health suffer if we have financial problems. My point is that what we do with our Fitness Account is very likely to affect the way other people see us. Overweight, bad posture and pale complexion are just a few of the signs that somebody is maxing out his Fitness Credit.

We all have the same start in the fitness Monopoly Game. We start with the same amount of capital and the same opportunities.

If we have been working out or if we were very lucky to be born with very good fitness genes, we might have a great line of fitness credit.

But as in the financial world, if you max out your fitness credit and pay back the minimum or have late or missed payments, you will ruin your fitness credit. If you do not keep up with your Give column and keep spending from your Take column of unhealthy decisions, your fitness credit will suffer no matter how healthy you have been and you will end up in bad health.

We have seen many great athletes end up in bad physical shape and even poor mental health. After they retired they completely changed their lifestyle and maxed out their fitness credit line.

It shouldn't be like this. And it won't be if we acknowledge the constant process of giving in and taking out from our health fitness account.

I have always believed that being healthy and happy can be achieved with simple daily exercises and balanced living. Staying in shape and enjoying activities that we love should not be hard. But one of the biggest challenges for people who try to follow fitness plans is to keep up with their routine and stay on track.

The comparison of financial and fitness planning is easy to follow because nearly everyone is aware of the importance of financial planning. To provide saving for our retirement is a strong motivator and often a source of a substantial amount of stress for many of us.

But many of us still do not recognize the importance of early planning to adopt a strategy that will let us retire in our best fitness and live a healthy and active life.

Although more and more people are hitting the gyms, trying to squeeze in a workout here and there, this still does not represent a real plan. The people I talk to have no plans for more than a couple of months ahead. When I ask some of the people at my gym, "What is your plan to stay healthy and fit for your retirement?" the answers I receive can be grouped in three categories:

1. I'll keep doing what I am doing now. People who exercise regularly and are in relatively good shape.

2. I'll hire a trainer to keep me healthy and happy (but I don't have the money for it right now).

3. I don't worry about my fitness after I retire. I will sleep in and play golf and drink beer. I don't need to be fit for that.

Let's look at those answers through our freshly opened Fitness Balance Sheet:

The first answer represents somebody who is building up his credit, constantly adding activities in his Give column and increasing his Health Credit Line. This book will help these people with guidelines to do even better by diversifying their Fitness Portfolio, learn new fitness activities and adopt lifestyles that guarantee they will stay healthy and happy.

People who give the second answer represent those of us who are not sure what to do, but realize the importance of staying fit and healthy over the long term and would prefer professional help. This is probably the biggest group.

The people who give the third answer believe that the money and wealth they have saved before retirement represent their health saving account. Unfortunately, this is rarely the case. The lifestyle suggested by the people that gave the third answer would quickly drain whatever health savings they have left.

I don't want to create another stress in your already busy everyday life. On the contrary, applying the 401 Fitness concept can help you find a simple way to organize and implement the most important plan in your life:

• Gain confidence and prepare your health and fitness for retirement.

• Put money in proper perspective with a holistic Fitness Balance Sheet.

• Take charge and invest in your physical autonomy.

During my years as a personal trainer I've talked to many clients and friends to ask them the same question: "Do you think you will be in a good health and fitness when you retire?"

Most people are very aware and concerned that their current lifestyle has no such guarantees. One of the most common concerns is that injuries will limit their activities and that slowly building weight will become a primary health issue.

By using well known and easily recognizable terms from finances and accounting, anyone can take a new approach to personal fitness and long-term planning for health.

When planning for your financial retirement, you need money that you can set aside or invest. For your fitness retirement, you will need money—but also time. You need to invest a piece of your personal time for every addition to your Give column.

Knowing where you want to be and having a realistic plan and budget is very important when you plan your financial investments. The same is valid when you are making your fitness wellness goals.

Chapter Six

Make Yourself a Priority

The key is not to prioritize what's on your schedule, but to schedule your priority.

— *Stephen R. Covey*

We all live by set of values that dictates where our priorities lie. Even if we do not recognize them, those values are the foundation of our goals, inspiration and everyday life. It seems logical that one of our top values should be "take care of yourself." It should be one of our top priorities because whatever we do, we will need our physical body to perform all the tasks we have in our busy lives. In the end, you are your longest commitment.

Thousands of years ago, when our predecessors were hunters and gatherers their entire lifestyle was based on that single priority—take care of yourself. Hunting, escaping from the predators, finding safe places for the night—all those activities that we also call "survival" are direct expressions of taking care of yourself. In those days, not following that priority would mean death.

Today we don't need to hunt or escape from predators or find a safe place to spend the night. We have jobs, air-conditioned offices and homes with flat screen TVs. Our business coaches help us to put our company's values and goals at the very top of our personal priorities. Every aspect of our life has its own logical demand for a place in that list. When was the last time somebody told you, "Make this a high priority," or, "This is a high priority project"?

Here is a simple exercise that will help you to compare priorities and see where they are in your list. The fitness accounting sheet that we created earlier comes in very handy in this exercise. Remember our fitness coins? Let's see where we are spending them.

Every time we pay with our hard-earned fitness coins, we deduct from our fitness savings. That "thing"—the activity that we are paying for with our fitness coins—is higher in our priority list than our health. Same goes for your time. Look where you are spending your time and you will find what activities are at the top of your priorities—no matter what goals you have written on your wall.

You are what you do every day.

It is normal if your values and priorities shift or change over time. Sometimes we get stuck with a value that no longer serves us. For example, when your kids are little they need you all the time and they are a top priority in your life. But when they grow up and leave home you can't keep that priority on top of your list anymore.

Your values shift naturally as you learn, meet new people or discover new ideas. You need to be aware of that process and respond with a lifestyle change based on your new top values. That is why we need to re-evaluate our values regularly and stay on top of them with our priorities.

There are many tools that can help you figure out what your top priorities are. I personally like Dr. John Demartini's value determination process—a free interactive tool on his web site: www.drdemartini.com.

It is an unfortunate fact that many people don't have time to exercise. Their own natural priority to take care of themselves has been pushed down the line by other "high priority" demands. Their personal health, fitness and happiness are waiting for some leftover time.

Even though we all have a subconscious feeling that we need to exercise, most of us do not have it in our schedules. And if we do, those precious time slots are the first to get pushed aside or eliminated by another higher priority.

When I meet new people socially and introduce myself as a personal trainer, the person I am talking with often tells me "I really need to start exercising, but I don't have the time." Sometimes they blame an injury in the past; or they moved and couldn't find a gym. I could write a book full of the excuses I have heard over the years. But the most common is, "I don't have time."

Most of the time when we think of exercising we tend to picture a gym or equipment and we also imagine spending hours of time. Of course, an hour of exercising would be great. But what if

you can't find that time slot? Or what if you
have it set in your schedule, but you keep
moving it around, rescheduling or canceling?
Sound familiar?

The main goal of this book is to help you
discover the missing foundations of movements
and activities in your lifestyle and help you
invest safe, small amounts of time to improve
your health and fitness in the long term.

Let's look again at our table with The Minimum
Requirements for Maintenance of the Ten
Foundations:

Minimum Requirements for Maintenance of the Ten Foundations

Daily	Breathing	Locom.	Hinge	Squat	Pull	Push	Rotations	Brain Fitness
	5 min.	5 min.	1 min.	1 min.	1min.	1 min.	1 min.	10 min.
Monthly	Social Fitness 1- 2 hours					Aqua Fitness 30-45 min		

If you look at all the movements that we should
do every day, they add up to 25 minutes. The
brain fitness exercise requires at least 10
minutes daily. Now if you have completed the
previous quiz and you have answered "I do
every day" in some categories, that means you
already covered that activity with your own
lifestyle. So, you can take that activity out and

you have only the remaining foundations to cover. For example, here is my typical daily routine:

- Wake up at 5 a.m.
- Yoga and Meditation: 20 minutes.
- Walk the dogs: 20 minutes.
- Creative writing.
- Teaching clients.
- Swim and sauna: 40-60 minutes.
- Lunch: 2-3 p.m.
- Nap: 20-30 minutes.
- Work with clients: 4-8 p.m.
- Dinner: 8-8:30 p.m.
- Go to bed with a book or TV: 9:30-10 p.m.
- Go to sleep: 11 p.m.

I can easily extract the following activities and match them with my Ten Foundations:

My morning yoga includes repetitive hinge, squat and pushing movements for 15 minutes followed by 5 minutes of meditation with breathing exercises. Walking the dogs takes me 20 minutes, then I write for 90 minutes.

When I work with clients, I strive to include at least seven of the foundational movements, and that often involves me demonstrating or doing the entire workout together with my client. To be on the safe side I would add 5 minutes of walking, running, squats, hinges, pullups, pushups, and various rotations. In the table below, you can see what foundations I have covered and what I need to work on.

	Breath	Loco	Hinge	Squat	Pull	Push	Rot	Brain	Social	Swim
Yoga and Meditation	5		5	5		5				
Walk the dogs		20								
Creative Writing								90		
Teaching AM		5	5	5	5	5	5			
Swimming										30
Teaching PM		5	5	5	5	5	5			
Total Time	**5**	**30**	**15**	**15**	**10**	**15**	**10**	**90**		**30**

In my case, I have all the foundations covered (except for social activities) in a single day.

The social activities requirement is 1-2 hours monthly. I belong to a group that meets for 3-4 hours every Wednesday. We play cards, chess and backgammon, so I have the social activity foundational minimum covered as well.

Even on days when I don't work with clients, I still have five or six foundations covered just with my morning routine.

Here is an empty table. Think about your typical day, and write down your activities on the left side, and put the times in minutes in the corresponding boxes under The Ten Foundations.

Your Activity	Breath	Loco	Hinge	Squat	Pull	Push	Rot	Brain	Social	Swim
Total Time										

Do you have empty columns? If so, you are not alone.

The purpose of this exercise is to help you see what foundations you have covered with your everyday routine. Those foundations that are not covered are the ones that you need to put as a top priority.

There are a couple of ways you can take care of those missing foundations. You can add exercises to your schedule or you can add activities to your lifestyle. Here are examples:

If you begin doing squats and push-ups every morning to cover those two foundational movements, you are adding exercises to your schedule.

The second option is to add an activity in your lifestyle that includes that missing foundation. For example, you can start taking the stairs instead the elevator, park further from the store so you can walk more, or squat or hinge when you tie your shoes.

You can use either of those options or both.

If you are one of those disciplined and consistent persons, adding exercises to your everyday life might be an easy fix for you. If you don't see any available time in your schedule for adding exercises, your best option is to add activities to your lifestyle.

I personally use both options. There are days when I don't walk the dogs or swim. To cover my foundations on those days I would do a workout using my TRX (Total Resistance eXercise) training. Other days when I know I will work long hours on my laptop, I opt to squat or sit on the floor, alternating positions as needed.

As long as you cover all your foundations, your health credit will grow, and your independent lifestyle will be more secure.

Not taking care of those missing or neglected foundations is like missing payments on your credit cards. It will eventually ruin your health credit.

In the next chapter, we will talk how to create short and effective blocks of exercises to cover your missing foundations.

Chapter Seven

One step, one breath at a time

Little by little, one travels far.

—*J. R. R. Tolkien*

The concept of breaking down long-term goals into small, doable steps is nothing new and has been proven to deliver its magic for centuries. Modern behavior specialists, coaches and therapists are using it every day to help their patients and clients.

In this chapter, I would like to suggest a few simple exercises and activities that can help you get started to cover your own *401 Fitness* foundations. Use the self-evaluating quiz to check what foundation needs your attention, then use the suggestions below to add an exercise or an activity to your lifestyle.

The *401 Fitness* five-minute foundation exercises:

1. Breathing.

That breath that you just took... that's a gift.

The benefits from performing the breathing exercises are immediate, and with discipline and consistency they turn into long term habits. Another thing I like about breathing exercises is that you can do them almost anywhere, at any time.

For the purpose of this book I suggest a very simple classification to help you choose an exercise to begin with.

- Breathing exercises that energize and stimulate.
- Breathing exercises that relax and calm you down.
- Breathing exercises for focus and concentration.

I encourage you to experiment with the length of time you inhale and exhale, and notice how it affects you. Some of the exercises that I suggest below already have "prescribed" lengths to inhale and exhale. But when you master the form, try different patterns.

This is your breath; one thing for which you should have full control and freedom. Use it.

Here is a very simple rule of thumb to determine how the way you breathe will affect you. If you inhale longer than you exhale, that breathing exercise will stimulate and energize you.

If the inhale is shorter than the exhale, it will relax and calm you down.

If you focus on equal breathing, in and out, it will help you concentrate.

Again, this is a very simplified way to look at the vast variety of breathing techniques and their benefits. I encourage you to keep exploring the magic of breathing on your own.

Before starting any of the following breathing exercises, do a mental scan for tightness in your body and try to relax. For example, we tend to "store" stress and tightness in our shoulders.

Relax your shoulders, let them drop down, and then begin with your breathing exercise.

Diaphragmatic (abdominal/belly) breathing:

With one hand on the chest and the other on the belly, take a deep breath in through the nose. Feel how your diaphragm inflates—the hand on your belly should move. The hand on your chest would eventually also move, but make sure the main movement is happening in your belly.

- Inhale through your nose for about two or three seconds.
- As you breathe out slowly, gently press on your belly hand to help the air out and promote the muscle memory of breathing "through" your belly
- Repeat.

Pursed-lips breathing:

- Breathe in through your nose for about two or three seconds.
- Breathe out very slowly through your mouth (like blowing out a candle), two to three times longer than you breathed in.
- Repeat.

Stimulating breathing:

- Inhale and exhale rapidly through your nose.

- Inhale and exhale are equal and as short as possible.

Balancing breath:

This exercise calms the nervous system, increases focus, and reduces stress.

- Inhale for a count of three, then exhale for a count of three.
- Inhale for a count of four, then exhale for a count of four.
- Inhale for a count of five, then exhale for a count of five.
- Inhale for a count of six, then exhale for a count of six.
- Repeat with the longest count you can handle.

I do this when I am already in, bed. It helps me to take my mind off any racing thoughts and calms me down.

Pick any of these simple techniques and use them daily. Create a habit to use breathing exercises when in traffic, at a red light, waiting on the phone, when you are stressed or nervous...

There are tons of breathing information online. When you feel comfortable using these techniques, look up my personal two favorite breathing exercises (these can be real espresso substitutes):

Nadi Shodhana: alternate nostril breathing.

Kapalabhati: "skull shining breath."

The *401 Fitness* Foundation Minimum for breathing exercises:

Pick any of the listed techniques and practice daily for at least five minutes without interruption.

2. Locomotion.

The locomotion exercises listed below are self-explanatory and simple enough to be performed by almost anybody without assistance. If you have problem with your knees or back, you should start with those that do not involve "flying moment" (such as hopping, leaping, running, jumping, galloping).

- Hopping: Spring from one foot and land on that same foot.
- Leaping: Spring from one foot and land on the other foot.
- Walking: Use your legs alternately to move from one place to another.
- Running: Like walking, but faster and with a flying moment.
- Jumping: Spring from both feet and land on both feet.
- Galloping: Run fast.
- Marching: Walk with regular steps of equal length.
- Skipping: Move lightly and quickly, from one foot to the other.
- Rolling: Moving or rolling on the floor, from side to side or forward and backward, or in combinations of both, while using natural body flexibility.
- Stepping: Step up or down, like when you are climbing stairs.
- Crawling: Moving in all directions using hands or elbows and feet or knees.

For your *401 Fitness* Foundation Minimum, pick one and perform it for one minute without interruption. For Walking, Marching and Running you can start with as little as 5 minutes a day. I suggest you start with walking if you have health problems that rule out the others on the list.

When you try all of these at least once, go ahead and try my personal favorite locomotor exercise: The Bear Walk.

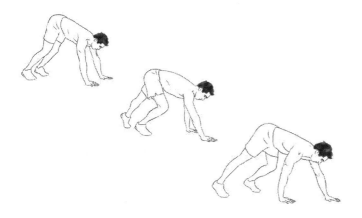

3. Hinge.

Hinge is all about good form!

Here are five form techniques to focus on:

- Sit back on your hips.
- Pull your belly in.
- Flatten your back (do not round your back at any time).
- Keep your knees soft.
- Look straight forward.

These are universal for all these hinge exercises:

- Hinge with a stick behind your back.
- **Good mornings.**
- Single-leg hinge to wall.
- Hip thrusts.

The exercises in this list can be done almost anywhere and do not require equipment. My personal favorite is not in this list—the Romanian Deadlift. I highly encourage you to learn the proper form with a trainer before trying it.

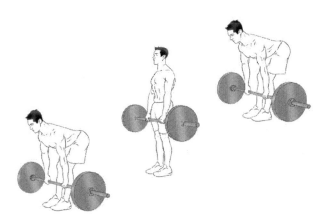

401 Fitness Foundation Minimum for hinge exercises: Pick one and perform it for one minute.

4. Squats.

I'll give you only two options here: partial squat and deep squat. If you have any health restrictions on deep squats, then begin with partial squats.

Form again is very important:

- Stand with your feet just over shoulder-width apart.

- Keep your back in a neutral position, and keep your knees centered over your feet.

- Slowly bend your knees, hips and ankles, lowering your butt to the bottom of your reach. Your feet should remain flat and your weight equally distributed on them.

- Push through your steady flat feet, keeping the knees from going out or in, and return to starting position.

- Inhale as you dip, exhale as you rise. Do not hold your breath at any time. When you master the form, try doing the squats with Pursed Leaps Breathing.

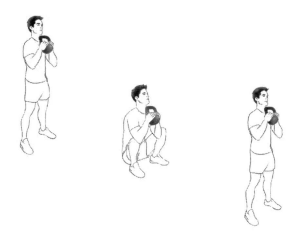

- For partial squats, choose the lowest chair or a step that you can squat to without compromising the form.

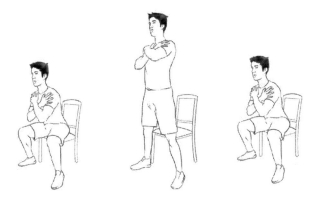

401 Fitness Foundation Minimum for squats: Squat as deep as you can for one minute. Use your body weight or hold a dumbbell as shown in the picture.

Tempo: Ten to fifteen repetitions per minute.

A great way to learn the form for deep squats is to perform them with the help of TRX (Total Resistance eXercise) system or any other suspension exercise system.

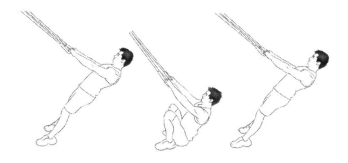

When you master the deep squat try the Pistol Squat—I am still working on that killer. Check the master calisthenics national known personal trainer Al Kavadlo's Instagram for inspiration.

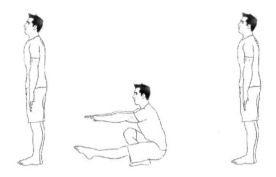

5. Rotation.

Torso rotation twist exercises are an important component of the Ten Fitness Foundations. These are also the most likely to be neglected in our regular daily routine—one more reason to make sure we cover the Foundation Minimum every day.

Here are illustrations of some of my favorite rotation exercises:

Bent-knee twist

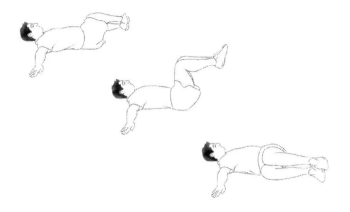

Russian Twist

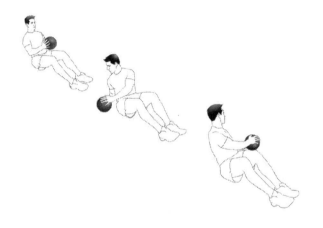

High and Low Twist

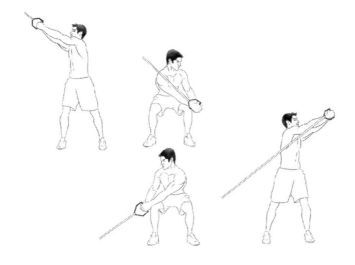

You can do all these without resistance and equipment, but for best results, use a medicine ball, resistance band or free weights.

401 Fitness Foundation Minimum for rotations: Do one of these for one minute.

Tempo: twenty to twenty-five repetitions per minute.

6. Push exercises.

These are bench presses, chest flies, dips, any type of shoulder presses, lateral or front raises, upright rows, etc. To keep it very simple I suggest only two exercises to cover the minimum of the push movement foundation.

Yes, this includes push-ups and dips. It can't get more simple than that. Modify your routine to follow the prescribed number of repetitions and tempo.

Push-ups: Engage your core and avoid your belly from sinking or your butt from sticking up. Lower all the way down and rest on the floor if you need to, but use the full range of movement from the bottom to the top instead of shortening the movement to just a few inches up and down.

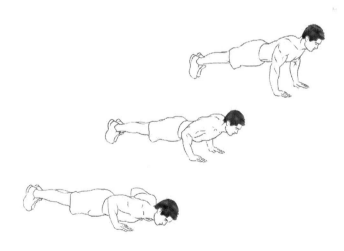

Dips: Chose a chair or other stable edge. Put your behind you on the surface with fingers facing forward; position your feet flat at shoulder width. You can modify the resistance by moving your feet closer or further. Lower your butt like you are trying to sit on the floor; keep your elbows pointed backward and your back close to the edge.

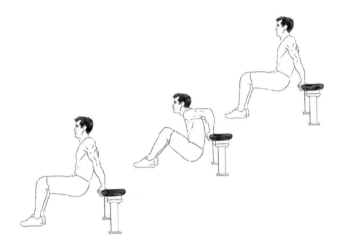

401 Fitness Foundation Minimum for push exercises:

Pick one or alternate both exercises for a total of one minute.

7. Pull exercises.

These are any bent-over or seated rows, reverse flies, pull ups, chin ups, pullovers, pulldowns, any type of bicep curls, etc.

116

My pick for covering this foundational movement is again very simple. I recommend pull-ups.

Use modifications as shown below to stay in between prescribed repetitions. My favorite is pull-ups using the TRX, alternating hand grips with palms facing out and in.

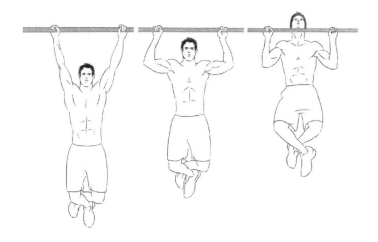

Another good pull exercise is the one-arm row. If you don't have a set of dumbbells or other weights, you can use a gallon of water or another household item. Keep your hips square and do not twist your torso. Move your elbow back and up until it passes the line of your back. Switch arms every ten to fifteen reps.

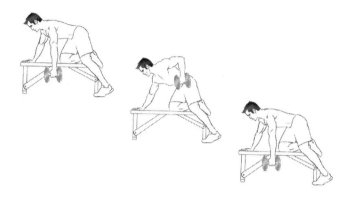

401 Fitness Foundation Minimum for pull exercises: **Perform one of these for one minute.**

8. Brain Fitness.

Our brains need to be stimulated constantly. Learning to stay present and pay attention to our surroundings is the most simple and natural way of providing learning material to our brain. That is how we have been using it for thousands of years. Paying attention and creating connections between things are still very beneficial for brain health. "Neurobic" exercises are like cross-training your brain. Exercises to strengthen brain function should offer novelty and challenge. "Almost any silly suggestion can work," says David Eagleman, PhD, neuroscientist, author and assistant professor at Baylor College of Medicine in Houston, Texas.

Here are examples that show how simple brain fitness can be:

- Brushing your teeth with your non-dominant hand.
- Switch seats at the table.
- Make connections with your nose (remember the smells on your way home).
- Make connections with your ears (listen to the outdoor noises and remember them).
- Use your fingers to recognize objects with your eyes closed.

The more senses you involve in your brain exercises the better.

Here are suggestions to help you start your brain fitness:

- Do the word puzzle, crossword or the Sudoku in your newspaper.
- Learn and play chess or backgammon.

There are so many ways to challenge your brain. But no, watching TV is not one of them. Read a book instead.

To cover your *401 Fitness* minimum, do any one of the above at least twenty minutes daily.

9. Social fitness.

> *"Right now, someone you haven't met is out there wondering what it would be like to meet someone like you."*
>
> —Unknown

Our social status, our friends and people we meet and spend time with are often more important for us than our health or the money we make. Another reason to include the social fitness in my Ten Foundations is because it is so easily manageable applying just two rules:

- Save and preserve.
- Invest and diversify.

We should preserve our existing relationships, and also identify and actively seek new people who would enrich our lives. Surround yourself with people who enjoy sharing meaningful, engaging conversations, and you never will feel alone. How many people can you call today to meet for coffee and just talk?

With our busy schedules, we often let our good friends drift away. Being an immigrant in this country, I quickly learned to appreciate the precious social value of my friends, colleagues and clients.

The minimum requirement to keep your social fitness in good shape is one to two hours monthly. There are many ways to get involved in groups and volunteer organizations, to meet new people. Here is my favorite simple "exercise" that I use:

Every week I try to meet with somebody that I haven't seen for at least a month. We get together for a coffee or beer or go for a walk. I call or text to check with that person and schedule a time to meet. I show appreciation for their time and express a sincere desire to reconnect and catch up.

When you meet, be on time and ask how much time your friend has. Here are five more tips to have in mind when meeting new people and even old friends:

- Smile.
- Make eye contact.
- Display positive body language.
- Ask great questions.
- Listen intently.

10. Aqua Fitness

If you can swim any style, congratulations! Swim! Use a snorkel, fins, paddles—anything to keep the practice interesting and challenging. My best personal discovery for swimming was the water-resistant iPod that enables me to listen to music or podcasts while swimming.

If you can't swim, I suggest you start with just walking in the water. Try different depths.

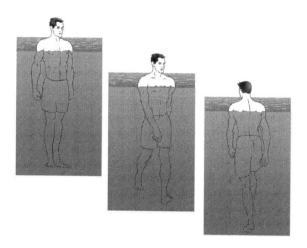

When you feel confident, learn to sink and float. The sinking and floating exercise will help you to develop your core and coordination as you maintain a prone position at all times. It will also boost your confidence in the water and it is the first step toward swimming. Here's how:

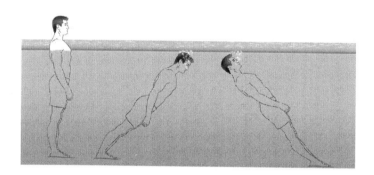

- Stand in the water up to your shoulders.

- Put your arms alongside as if they are glued to your body.
- Take a breath and start tilting forward, keeping your body straight and feet glued to the bottom of the pool.
- Try this forward, backward and even sideways. Notice how your body floats and sinks.
- Next stage: Do the same, but this time when you fall forward and your face is in the water, start blowing out some air and let your feet leave the bottom. The remaining air in your lungs will keep you afloat. You will float forward for a little. Try to relax and enjoy that feeling of lightness.
- When you get comfortable with floating forward, try it backward as well.

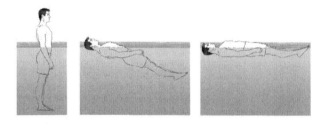

- Make sure you are comfortable with the floating exercises before trying to sink. To sink, just continue blowing your air out until you feel that buoyance disappears and your body slowly sinks.

- As you sink to the bottom, lay back and try to relax and enjoy the new perceptions.
- When you can't hold your breath any longer, slowly bring your feet under you and stand up (remember, you are still in shoulder-deep water).

Floating and sinking doesn't require motor skills or muscle memory. You need only confidence and relaxation.

The *401 Fitness* Foundation Minimum for aqua fitness: If you can swim, by all means enjoy this unique and natural full-body activity. If you can't swim, start with walking, floating and sinking exercises. Practice at least thirty to forty-five minutes every month.

All the exercises suggested in this chapter can be done with or without equipment by any beginner. If you feel that you can do harder variations or more difficult exercises, go for it. My goal was to present exercises that everybody will be able to start with and cover their missing foundations.

Chapter Eight

Make the Most of Every Step

You need to stay active. My grandmother started walking five miles a day when she was 60. She is 97 now and we don't know where the hell she is.

— *Ellen DeGeneres*

Mama Pepe is the sister-in-law to my wife's dad. I am not even sure if this description is proper, but it doesn't matter. For everyone who knows her she is Mama Pepe—she has become an institution. Her amazing personality makes interacting with four generations of relatives and friends so easy that all of us enjoy her company and feel the need to stay in touch.

One thing that I have learned from her is that there can't be "an empty course." If, for example, we are having dinner at the table at home and one of us needs to go to the kitchen for some reason, she would give him something to carry to the kitchen—an empty plate that is no longer needed, a bottle to put away, or something else... just something to add more value to that kitchen trip.

We often laugh about that in our family, but I recently realized how many times in my day I am using that "no empty course" approach to manage my day and free up time for myself. If I need to go to the basement or the garage for something, I would first look around to see if I can take something that needs to be there. If I am about to drive longer than fifteen minutes I always put a podcast or an audio book on. Put things where they belong, clear your desk and spend just a minute to tidy up—and pretty soon you will find that you have freed up an hour for yourself.

Finding ways to make every activity even more efficient has become a habit of mine. Freeing minutes here and there can give us that extra time for meditation or stretching that we weren't able to fit in.

Lack of time is probably the most often used excuse to not take care of ourselves. We all have ways to become more efficient and free up time for ourselves. Optimizing everyday activities and combining trips has become part of my life. A big part of this book I have written in a deep squat or sitting and stretching on the floor. So don't mind if you notice my wording is cramping or my sentence being stiff here and there, it was probably the early morning stretch and writing.

If it only takes five minutes, do it now

In this chapter I would like to offer you a micro workout, that would help you to cover the Minimum Daily Requirements of your Fitness Foundations.

The routine represents the very minimum of physical activities that you must have in your everyday life. If you do not have five or six minutes for yourself, you are doing something wrong.

The idea behind the micro workout is to provide stand-alone block of five- or six-minute exercises using the foundational movements.

You won't see a specific exercise for your brain in the list, but here is how you can actually exercise your brain for the entire time of the 401 MicroFit. Try and do one or more of the following:

- Listen to music and try to remember the order of the songs, the words, or what song was playing when each exercise started.

- Do the entire workout with bare feet or with gloves and notice how it feels.
- Do the workout with one or both eyes closed.

These simple challenges will engage your brain while you exercise.

If you have time to go to a gym, you should do more work. Here I am suggesting exercises for those who don't have time to go to a gym and do not have access to equipment. The only thing you need is to set aside five-six minutes of your time and show up.

401 MicroFit: a six-minute routine

Set your timer to beep every sixty seconds. If you do not have a timer, aim for the prescribed number of repetitions next to the exercises, and move to the next exercise when you reach your maximum.

Begin with five deep, energizing abdominal breaths.

Inhale through your nose for a count of four or five. Let the air fill in your belly.

Exhale powerfully trough your mouth for a count of three. Press gently with one hand on your belly to help the air go out.

Start your six-minute timer now.

Perform each of the following exercises for one minute or do the prescribed repetitions, limit your rest time between to 15-20 seconds or five deep breaths:

Squats (bodyweight deep squats or squat to a chair): 20 reps or as many as you can do with good form for 60 seconds

Good mornings (hinge): 20 reps or as many as you can do with good form for 60 seconds

Bend over row (use rubber bands, or weights): 10 reps or as many as you can do with good form for 60 seconds

Caterpillars forward on hands then feet follow: 5 reps or as many as you can do with good form for 60 seconds

Bicycle Crunches: 20 reps or as many as you can do with good form for 60 seconds

Push-ups: 10 reps or as many as you can do with good form for 60 seconds

Modify any of the exercises and use the resistance so you can perform the original movement with a good form.

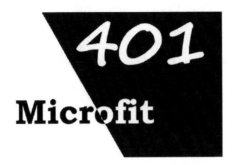

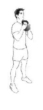 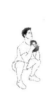 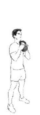 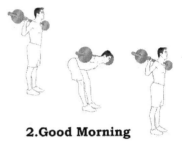

1.Deep Squat   **2.Good Morning**

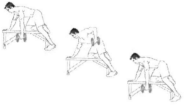 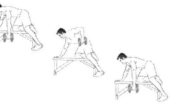   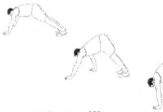

3.Bent Over Dumbbell Row   **4.Caterpillar**

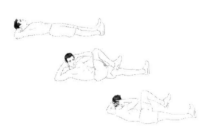   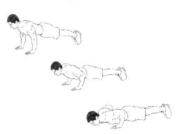

5.Bicycle Crunches   **6.Push Ups**

132

Congratulations, you just invested six minutes in your health.

If you have few more minutes to spare, I highly recommend you spend some time on the floor after finishing the push-ups. Stretch out on your back and do the child pose or simply close your eyes and breathe. Those quite moments are like an hour at the spa for your brain.

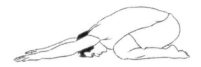

How does doing these exercises feel? Was it surprisingly challenging, or maybe too easy?

The micro routine above is the very minimum of physical activities everyone should do to stay on top of their fitness account.

It is like paying just the minimum to your credit card. It does not pay off your balance, but at least keeps your credit score good.

I know people who would not be able to do these exercises without modifications. If you feel the same, please, by all means contact me and I'll be more than happy to suggest alternative exercises and proper modifications.

Let's now compare the six-minute micro routine with the minimum requirements for the Ten Foundations.

Daily Requirements for The Ten Foundations:

Breathing Work:

Five minutes of uninterrupted practice.

Locomotion:

Five minutes of uninterrupted practice.

Hinge:

One minute of uninterrupted activity that includes those movements.

Squat:

One minute of uninterrupted activity that includes that movement.

Rotation:

One minute of uninterrupted activity that includes those movement.

Push:

One minute of uninterrupted activity that includes those movements

Pull:

One minute of uninterrupted activity that includes those movements.

Brain Fitness:

Ten minutes of uninterrupted activity.

Monthly Requirements for The Ten Foundations

Social Fitness: One to two hours of engagement.

Aqua Fitness: Thirty to forty-five minutes.

Minimum Requirements for Maintenance of the Ten Foundations

Daily	Breathing	Locom.	Hinge	Squat	Pull	Push	Rotations	Brain Fitness
	5 min.	5 min.	1 min.	1 min.	1min.	1 min.	1 min.	10 min.
Monthly	Social Fitness 1- 2 hours				Aqua Fitness 30-45 min			

As you can see, if we add up the times for the daily requirements we will end up with 15 minutes for the first seven, plus ten minutes for brain fitness. With the six minutes of 401MicroFit workout we covered very important part of the daily requirements. The Hinge, Squat, Pull, Push and Rotation movements often get neglected in our everyday routine.

Here is an important point: If the quiz in Chapter Three showed that your lifestyle does not cover any of the Ten Foundations, you need to find time to do the 401MicroFit workout at least once per day and add ten minutes of brain fitness to your routine.

People who go to work, do their own shopping, gardening and housekeeping would find out from the quiz that they already have covered a lot of the minimal daily requirements for physical activities, the remaining will be covered with 401MicroFit. Think about The 401MicroFit as a stand-alone mini workout, that you can do anywhere and on your own.

It is easier to set a side 6 minutes time once a day and stay on the top of your Ten Foundations.

For some time now, my wife and I wear these smart devices that count steps along with other cool features. I was very surprised when we compared our steps at the end of the first day. My wife had over 10,000 steps and I had about half as many. My wife is an accountant and she is supposed to spend a lot of time behind her desk. I move around a lot and often walk and run with my clients.

What I discovered, after looking into this, was that despite my "active" lifestyle, I actually sit a lot. Of course, a big chunk of the difference between our steps was coming from the fact that my steps are almost twice as long as my wife's. But I also discovered that I spend a lot of my day driving between clients and sitting in my car. At the same time, my wife was adding up steps walking to her co-worker's desk, climbing stairs in her office and making trips to the printer and the office kitchen.

Do not underestimate the opportunities to move that your day offers to you. You can add exercises to your schedule, but that's not very easy if your schedule is already full. Or you can add or change your routine to gain more activities, such as parking farther away from the store to give you those extra steps that you need after a long day of sitting.

The energy that your body needs just for functioning is called basal metabolic rate, or BMR. If you choose a lifestyle that requires constantly moving and avoid long sitting you increase your BMR and enjoy the benefits of burning more calories without even noticing it.

Look around and find ways to move and do more, not less. Use that "no empty course" wisdom of Mama Pepe. I am sure she wouldn't mind to keep you busy the way she always does for us.

Chapter Nine

Get the Most from Your Trainer

Plans are only good intentions unless they immediately degenerate into hard work.

— *Peter Drucker*

I met Jon few years ago. He was dating a very active and fit lady. They were making plans to get married and had just started working out together. For a couple of months before the wedding they would wake up early and exercise with me. I could see how his fiancé was trying hard to get Jon motivated and help him get in shape.

At the beginning Jon was consistent and showed up. But after a few weeks that changed. He began to show up late most of the time or not show up at all. Many mornings I ended up working out with his future wife while he was still sleeping.

After the wedding Jon started finding more and more excuses and kept missing workouts until one day he just completely dropped the training. His wife continued to work out with me for a few months, even though she didn't need my help because she already had an active lifestyle with exercise classes and sports events planned well ahead.

A year after the wedding they divorced. Jon called, and we met at a restaurant. He was having a hard time dealing with his emotions and I felt really bad for him. He wanted to start working out again. He said he would do everything I asked him to do on his own. I told him that this might not work because in the past he wasn't able to demonstrate self-motivation and discipline, even when I was ringing his doorbell, right there in person to help him out.

Jon is a very nice guy, so I reluctantly agreed to help him with his plan, knowing in my heart that it probably wouldn't work. I hoped he could use his emotional crisis as a good motivator to push him into keeping a healthier daily routine. I made him promise that he would follow the plan and stay on track. So I designed a program with exercises that I knew he could do on his own, and we agreed that he would text me every morning when he finished exercising.

If you are guessing that it didn't happen, you are right! He never texted me after exercising and when I texted him to ask about it he would respond very shortly that he did the exercises and they went well. Yes, I had the same feeling you are probably having right now—that Jon was not doing anything. After two weeks, he stopped responding to my texts.

Why am I am telling you this story?

Because knowing and honestly admitting your weaknesses is a very important step when you are making plans. Even if we have the support of our family and friends, in the end it is up to us to step up and do our job. Nobody can exercise for us.

It might be better to have extra help, especially at the beginning, until you build up a habit. But many people overestimate their own discipline and motivation. Making the same mistakes regardless of what previous experience has taught you will lead to the same results from the past.

And no matter how good your support group is, no matter how much help you plan to get, you still need to do your part and *show up.*

Remember: There is no way to get away with *not* showing up for your personal fitness investment. There is no way that your spouse or your trainer can do the work for you.

The good news is that the more you show up and do your part, the easier it gets. With time, you will need less and less help and motivation from outside.

This is important for our fitness planning. Imagine that after completing an evaluation with your trainer you conclude that you need to start working out every day. Your monthly budget can't afford paying a trainer to be there all the time. So how will you make this happen?

Use your trainer as a rocket to lift you to the place you can fly alone. Repeat that process every time when you set new "altitude" goals.

Here is an example.

Let's say that after evaluating your fitness and health you decide that you need to lose twenty pounds. With this goal in mind you meet with a trainer.

Your health is of highest value for you and you searched for the best trainer in your area, so it is not a surprise that this trainer comes with a high price and has many clients ahead of you on his schedule. But you arrange a meeting. Good trainers do the first session at no charge to get to know you and go over the plan.

After listening to your goals and performing the usual assessments, the trainer suggests a fitness plan that requires you to exercise for an hour, three times a week. Everything is pretty standard so far, right? But now you have to be smart and careful with your budget.

The most expensive thing in your training is time with your trainer. Your goal is to optimize your spending and still get the benefits from working with the best trainer in your area.

But for many years I have witnessed people starting on and dropping off programs, diets, health regimens and all kinds of fitness plans because they didn't plan or consider all the important factors of their training.

I put these factors in two main groups:

Outside factors:

- Support (family, friends, co-workers, etc.).
- Quality of professional help (trainer's experience, knowledge and abilities).

Inside factors:

- Motivation (why you want to exercise) - A
- Time you have available for exercising on your own - B
- Ability to perform exercises in a good form - C
- Discipline and consistency - D
- Budget – E
- Frequency of exercising per week - F

The stronger your A, B, C and D are, the less E and F you will need.

Here are few strategy examples of how this can be applied in training plans:

Strategy	Duration	Frequency	Total Sessions	Cost Per Session	Total Budget
Beginner A	8 weeks	3,3,3,3 x 2	24	$80	$1,920
Beginner B	8 weeks	3,2,1,0 x 2	12	$85	$1,020
Advanced	8 weeks	2,1,1,1 x 2	10	$90	$900
Expert	8 weeks	1,0,1,0 x 2	4	$125	$500

Strategy	Apply this strategy if:
Beginner A	• You are very new to fitness training with zero or little experience. • You have an injury, or you are recovering from one. • You need to build your discipline and consistency.
Beginner B	• You are a beginner with some experience. • You can follow a printed exercise program.
Advanced	• You can demonstrate good form with all the exercises from the program. • You have demonstrated that you can be effective on your own following a program and even modifying it when needed.
Expert	• You have great form and ability to follow printed programs and modify or exchange exercises. • You demonstrate discipline and consistency.

All the strategies are based on an eight-week plan. The rates in these examples represent the current rates (2018) for the best fitness trainers in the Cincinnati, Ohio area. It is a standard practice the cost per session to drop if you buy a package with multiple sessions.

In my practice I use customized variations of these strategies, and I also combine them with the resources of my online training center. In real life, when you take out the time you are gone on vacation, travel, or you are sick or not able to work out, you might have forty or forty-five weeks available in any given year. This is actually not a bad number, if you use a smart strategy for your training.

Here are two more examples of time and budget distribution depending on your level:

If you start working out following the first strategy—such as Beginner A for your first eight weeks—you should be able to "graduate" to Beginner B and work you way up to Advanced. Then you can continue until you become an Expert. At that point you should be able to continue on your own using professional help only when you need to change a routine or need help with specific exercise form or a fitness assessment. The first strategy—Beginner A—is suitable for somebody that has zero or very little experience working out. If you are not sure where to start, always start as a Beginner or a step lower than you think you should be.

No matter how strong the outside factors are, you cannot just rely on them for your success. Training is not a service that you can just pay for and then passively wait for a miracle to happen. You need to do more on your own than you do with your trainer if you want to accomplish your goals.

Here are some relations between the inside factors that I have observed when working with students and clients:

1. The stronger your motivation is, the more likely you are to follow the program and get the results.
2. The more time you set aside to exercise with your trainer and also on your own, the faster you will see results and become independent.
3. The more disciplined and consistent you are, the more effective your plan will be for you, and the faster you will build self-discipline and autonomy.
4. The bigger your budget is, the more tools and activities your trainer can expose you to.

5. The more frequent you exercise in a week, the faster you will be on your own

People often overlook these factors or only consider budget or time. That leads to paying for something that might not fit, like buying shoes just for their color.

Good personal trainers use their intuition, knowledge and experience to design a fitness plan that will reflect all the above factors and help you create your own support group among your family and friends. Good trainers also encourage you to explore and try different fitness classes, trainers and teachers. This is how you will become independent and sustainable in your training, and that is the best way to adopt a healthy lifestyle. There is no sustainability in your training if it relies only on outside factors (trainers, family, friends).

One of the best rewards in my line of work is when a client decides to try new things, such as starting a fitness or yoga class or working out on their own. Those are signs that my "rocket" has played its role, providing the altitude and speed my clients need to fly on their own.

Fitness **Smart Strategy**

Outside factors:

Make a list of friends, family, and co-workers who can motivate and support you. Share with them your goals and progress and ask them to keep you accountable.

Make a list of the five best personal trainers available in your area and meet them in person to decide whom to hire. Base your decision on the trainer's experience working with people who have goals like yours. Look for trainers who will provide the tools to track your progress and who take a holistic approach to your problem— such as a nutrition plan or mind/body exercises to keep your stress low.

Inside factors:

Sit down and evaluate your inside factors on a piece of paper.

149

A) Your personal Motivation for exercising is the fuel for your journey. Get to the roots of it to understand your strengths.

B) Look closely at your daily, weekly and monthly **Time** schedules and planed activities. Discover the available times slots for exercises, and make sure you are not creating conflicts, because you want to create a sustainable lifestyle, not just a temporary fix.

C) Pick an exercise that you never did and see if you have the **Ability** to do it with good form, following written or video directions. Use a mirror to check your form. Work on developing this skill, to increase the effectiveness of your workout and decrease your budget.

D) Make an honest evaluation of your **Discipline** and ability to follow a plan. List examples that demonstrate your self-discipline from previous experiences. Ask your family and friends to evaluate your discipline on a scale from 1 to 10 and compare that with your own evaluation.

E) Think about how much **Budget** you can afford for a period from sixteen to forty-eight weeks. The more experience you have, the less time you need. Short time "fixes" to "get in shape for a week" don't work, because you wind up back at the same starting point year after year.

F) **Frequency** is very important because it distributes not only the load and time of the exercises, but also the load to your schedule and budget. Here are some frequency suggestions to consider when working on your plan:

Frequency	Experience	Goals
Daily	Beginner/Low Self-Discipline	Establish moving foundations, build habits, lose weight
Every Other Day	Beginner	Build strength, lose weight
Once a week	Advanced	Maintenance
Once every other week	Advanced	Specific strength or skills
Once a month	Expert	Maintenance

The *401 Fitness* Smart Strategy allows anybody to plan, begin and follow through on a journey to better health and an independent, active life.

Chapter Ten

Make it Easy, Start Small

You will never change your life until you change something that you do daily. The secret of your success is found in your daily routine.

— John C. Maxwell

Adopting healthy habits is the only way I know that works toward better health.

Every morning at 5, I open my eyes just a few minutes before my alarm goes off. It is not easy to leave the warm bed, especially on a cold dark morning. There is always this voice in the back of my head telling me that it is still very early, it is very dark and cold outside, and I should go back to sleep for "just a couple more minutes." I admit that many times I listened to that convincing voice and went back to sleep.

But a long time ago I came to the realization that early mornings are my most productive time. It is also easy for me to fit a quick workout

152

in the few extra hours at the beginning of my day. So, I intentionally decided to build a habit to get up early and do my morning exercise routine and creative work first thing. Here are some interesting things that I discovered in those early mornings, that I am sure happen only to me:

- The cold water is extra cold.
- The quieter you are trying to be the more noise you make.
- Espresso machines break only in the morning.
- Cats are sassy.
- Dogs are lazy.
- If you look just for a second at your phone, your time evaporates in emails and texts and suddenly it is already time to leave home.

There have been times that it feels like the whole universe has something against my early morning routines.

Here are some of my secret weapons to push through those obstacles and create a habit:

Start with a simple **doable task**. Don't try to change your whole life. Pick the smallest doable thing you can repeat and you are in the game. It is a journey. I created the *401MicroFit* Routine for that purpose, but, if it is too much, modify the exercises or cut it short.

Look at your calendar and plan an available and convenient time for your commitment. You do not want to start building a habit that will mess up your entire schedule. Make sure there are no planned events that will be in a conflict. Be realistic: Don't start a healthy eating habit just before Thanksgiving. There is a notion that a habit is created in twenty-one days. I prefer to aim for four weeks or a month. Pick a month from your calendar and make a **daily commitment for thirty days.**

To create a habit, you need to **do it every day,** preferably at the same time and place. You will have a harder time creating your healthy habit if you do the activity just once or twice a week. It is easier to adopt a habit if you consistently repeat it over and over at the **same place and at the same time** every day. That will reinforce the patterns of your environment and they will become your cues to do the activity.

Plan **reminders and tools that will keep you on track**. Use your phone or watch alarm, print out a check list or ask a friend or family member to remind you and keep you motivated.

Keep in mind that it won't be easy and there will be some problems down the road but stay consistent and trust the process. There were days when I stayed in bed longer and missed my morning fitness routine. **Accept that you are not perfect all the time but remember the benefits.** Picture yourself with the benefits of making the change.

I noticed that if I just look at my phone in the morning it is very likely I'll end up spending my precious creative hours by responding to texts or e-mails that actually can wait. So, now I do not even look at my phone in the morning. I keep it in a non-disturb mode and it is not even on my desk. **Remove obstacles** and temptations that get in your way.

Surround yourself with people who represent the model of your desired behavior. Spend time in circles where your values and motivations are shared, but remember that at the end it is *you* doing this for your own benefit, not for somebody's approval.

And finally, I have a "secret" hack. It is a simple thing that works for me and helps me to get up and keep up with my morning routine. It is something like a mantra that I repeat, to help me start and keep moving even on the darkest and coldest mornings. I repeat to myself, "One foot after the other, one foot after the other." I begin with the smallest movements and keep repeating it until I build the momentum to follow my routine. As simple as it is, it works like a miracle.

When it is dark and cold, and my inner voice is trying to keep me in the warm and cozy bed, I tell myself, "One foot after the other." I reach out under the blanket with my bare foot to the cold floor: "One foot after the other." I bring my other leg out from under the covers and to the floor: "One foot after the other." I open my eyes: "One foot after the other." I stretch, still sitting in bed: "One foot after the other." I stand up and move to the bathroom: "One foot after the other." The cold water is really cold again: "One foot after the other."

I think the first step is the most important one when it comes to creating habits. It can be a long journey, but everything happens after we take that first step.

Breaking down your first step to a very doable and simple task is very important for your success. Make as many first steps as you need to start moving and create momentum for the second step.

There is no such thing as a very little first step. All first steps are huge, because they give us the direction and create the momentum of change. If you can't make your first step, that only means that you need to break it further down. Make it as simple and as doable as possible.

The first step is not about distance, it is about the direction and the momentum that you need for the second, the third and all the following steps of your journey.

The main idea behind this book is to give a different perspective on what working out would look like, even if you think that you have all the excuses in the world not to exercise.

Understanding that there is no such thing like doing too little will help you create your very important first step. The Ten Foundations represent my view of the minimum of activities and movements that our human body and brain needs every day if we want to stay mobile, active and happy.

Here are few suggestions to apply to build your very own fitness and health wealth:

Use the self-evaluation quiz or get help from a professional to determine which of the Ten Foundations you need to work on.

Then use the exercises presented in this book— the *401 MicroFit* Routine—to build up your fitness credit.

When you establish your fitness foundations, invest time to explore and challenge your body and mind with your choice of branded activities.

If you need to work with a trainer, use the *401 Fitness Smart Budget Strategy* tool to create your custom fitness plan.

Create habits. Find your mantra that makes you move when it is hard to take the first step and follow your plan. It takes time to create a habit, but the reward is your own fitness and health wealth.

The principles of *401 Fitness* are simple, easy to integrate and they work for anyone and everyone. We were all designed to be healthy and happy. Building upon your Ten Foundation movements and activities will enable you to experience your inherent abilities to heal, recover and evolve.

One foot after the other.

Acknowledgements

This book would not have been possible without the help and inspiration of many people who encouraged me to share my fitness philosophy in *401 Fitness*. I would like to give special thanks to the following:

My best friend, soulmate and wife, Dani: Thank you for believing in me and being the anchor of my kite!

My son Mitko, for all the support, inspiration and the great time we spend together that means more to me than anything!

My clients, for trusting my work, forgiving my mistakes when I count their reps, dealing with my heavy accent, and always paying on time. Seriously, you guys rock!

My friends and family in Bulgaria, US, Canada, Germany, Belgium, England, Netherlands and the rest of the world. Thank you for all the support, laughter, good food and hospitality. Looking forward to spending more time together.

For Mom: Mom, I promise I'll translate the book for you in Bulgarian and we will do the *401 MicroFit* together.

Peter Bronson: Thank you for encouraging and coaching me to write. A lot of my motivation came after you told me that my writing was "good stuff."

Welcome to My Village

It takes a village to raise a child.

African proverb.

This wisdom exists in different forms in many African languages. The basic meaning is that raising a child is a communal effort. The responsibility for raising a child is shared with the larger family (sometimes called the extended family). Everyone in the family participates, especially with older children—aunts, uncles, grandparents, even cousins. And the wider community gets involved, such as neighbors and friends.

Nobody is born with knowledge and experience. The unique ability to learn, interpret and apply knowledge has been the leading force of human progress.

Every day we are exposed to hundreds of simple and complex experiences, and it is up to each of us to decide which to choose as valuable lessons. Some lessons we seek and even pay for, others will hit us from the blue and we might

162

not be ready to understand them. Keeping our minds open and staying hungry for new experiences tremendously widens our "village" of sources for learning and increases our chances to make better lifestyle choices.

Some people are trained to give lessons; others are born teachers. We expect to learn from teachers, but we are also exposed to a great variety of regular people who can enrich us with their own unique experiences and knowledge.

Every person carries lessons to pass along. We just need to stay curious, listen, and pick those lessons that will make us better.

"<u>The village</u>" is my virtual collective community of professional and amateur teachers that I constantly learn from.

Meet some of my teachers, trainers and important "villagers" who have influenced me with priceless lessons, inspiration and motivation. Some I have not met in person; others I have the privilege to call friends. My village is growing with every blog or book I read, every podcast I listen to or even a neat Instagram post. Who is in your village?

Made in the USA
Columbia, SC
07 September 2023

22488915R00093